D1243594

NUTRITION in EXERCISE and SPORT

Edited by Ira Wolinsky and James F. Hickson, Jr.

Published Titles

Exercise and Disease,
Ronald R. Watson and Marianne Eisinger
Nutrients as Ergogenic Aids for Sports and Exercise,
Luke Bucci
Nutrition in Exercise and Sport, Second Edition,
Ira Wolinsky and James F. Hickson, Jr.
Nutrition Applied to Injury Rehabilitation and Sports Medicine,
Luke Bucci
Nutrition for the Recreational Athlete,
Catherine G.R. Jackson

NUTRITION in EXERCISE and SPORT

Edited by Ira Wolinsky

Published Titles

Sports Nutrition: Minerals and Electrolytes,
Constance V. Kies and Judy A. Driskell
Nutrition, Physical Activity, and Health in Early Life:
Studies in Preschool Children,
Jana Parizkova
Exercise and Immune Function,
Laurie Hoffman-Goetz
Body Fluid Balance: Exercise and Sport,
E.R. Buskirk and S. Puhl
Nutrition and the Female Athlete,
Jaime S. Ruud
Sports Nutrition: Vitamins and Trace Elements,
Ira Wolinsky and Judy A. Driskell
Amino Acids and Proteins for the Athlete—The Anabolic Edge,
Mauro G. DiPasquale
Nutrition in Exercise and Sport, Third Edition,
Ira Wolinsky

Published Titles (continued)

Gender Differences in Metabolism: Practical and Nutritional Implications, Mark Tarnopolsky

Macroelements, Water, and Electrolytes in Sports Nutrition, Judy A. Driskell and Ira Wolinsky

Sports Nutrition, Judy A. Driskell

Energy-Yielding Macronutrients and Energy Metabolism in Sports Nutrition, Judy A. Driskell and Ira Wolinsky

Nutrition and Exercise Immunology, David C. Nieman and Bente Klarlund Pedersen

NUTRITION in EXERCISE and SPORT

Edited by Ira Wolinsky

Forthcoming Titles

High Performance Nutrition: Diets and Supplements for the Competitive Athlete, Mauro DiPasquale

Nutrition and the Strength Athlete, Catherine R. Jackson

Sports Drinks: Basic Science and Practical Aspects, Ronald Maughan and Robert Murry

Nutritional Applications in Exercise and Sport, Ira Wolinsky and Judy Driskell

Nutrients as Ergogenic Aids for Sports and Exercise, Second Edition, Luke R. Bucci

NUTRITION *and* EXERCISE IMMUNOLOGY

David C. Nieman
Bente Klarlund Pedersen

CRC Press
Boca Raton   London   New York   Washington, D.C.

Library of Congress Cataloging-in-Publication Data

Nutrition and exercise immunology / edited by David C. Nieman, Bente K. Pedersen.
    p.cm -- (Nutrition in exercise and sport)
Includes bibliographical references and index.
ISBN 0-8493-0741-4 (alk. paper)
1. Exercise--Immunological aspects. 2. Nutrition. I. Nieman, David C., 1950-II
Pedersen, Bente Klarlund, 1956-III. Series.
QP301.N875 2000
616.07'9--dc21   00-021954
                                                                                 CIP

© 2000 by CRC Press LLC

No claim to original U.S. Government works
International Standard Book Number 0-8493-0741-4
Library of Congress Card Number 00-021954
Printed in the United States of America 1 2 3 4 5 6 7 8 9 0
Printed on acid-free paper

Series Preface

The CRC series *Nutrition in Exercise and Sport* provides a setting for in-depth exploration of the many and varied aspects of nutrition and exercise, including sports. The topic of exercise and sports nutrition has been a focus of research among scientists since the 1960s, and the healthful benefits of good nutrition and exercise have been appreciated. As our knowledge expands, it will be necessary to remember that there must be a range of diets and exercise regimes that will support excellent physical condition and performance. There is not a single diet–exercise treatment that can be the common denominator, or the single formula for health, or a panacea for performance.

This series is dedicated to providing a stage upon which to explore these issues. Each volume provides a detailed and scholarly examination of some aspect of the topic. Contributors from bona fide areas of nutrition and physical activity, including sports and the controversial, are welcome.

We welcome the authoritative contribution *Nutrition and Exercise Immunology*, edited by David C. Nieman and Bente Klarlund Pederson. This volume will have interest and application in several important fields.

Ira Wolinsky, Ph.D.
Series Editor

Preface

The immune system is a remarkably adaptive defense entity that is able to generate an enormous variety of cells and molecules capable of recognizing and eliminating a limitless variety of foreign invaders. Nutrition impacts the development of the immune system, both in the growing fetus and in the early months of life. Nutrients are also necessary for the immune response to pathogens so cells can divide and produce antibodies and cytokines. Many enzymes in immune cells require the presence of micronutrients, and critical roles have been defined for zinc, iron, copper, selenium, vitamins A, B_6, C, and E in the maintenance of optimum immune function.

The earliest research on nutrition and immune function focused on malnutrition. It has long been known that malnourished children have a high risk of severe and life-threatening infections. Protein-energy malnutrition adversely affects virtually all components of the immune system. Current investigation has centered on the role of specific nutrient deficiencies and nutrient supplements on immune function in a wide variety of human subjects including the elderly, children and adults from developing countries, human immunodeficiency virus (HIV)-infected patients, eating-disorder patients, and healthy adults.

A burgeoning area of scientific endeavor is the influence of nutrition on the immune changes that occur with acute and chronic exercise. Many components of the immune system exhibit change after prolonged heavy exertion, indicating that the immune system is stressed, albeit transiently, following prolonged endurance exercise. There is evidence that risk of respiratory infection may be increased when the endurance athlete goes through repeated cycles of heavy exertion, has been exposed to novel pathogens, or experienced other stressors to the immune system including lack of sleep, severe mental stress, malnutrition, or weight loss. Although endurance athletes can lower infection risk through various hygienic practices, they must undergo intense training cycles to compete successfully. As a result of these data, interest in nutrition and various nutrient supplements with the potential to influence exercise-induced alterations in immunosurveillance has grown. In this volume, leading investigators from around the world review the link between nutrition and immune function, with special application to athletic endeavor.

David C. Nieman, Dr.PH., FACSM

Bente K. Pedersen, Ph.D.

About the Editors

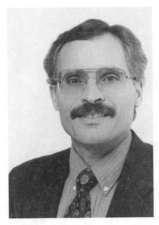

David C. Nieman, Dr.PH., FACSM, graduated from Loma Linda University in 1984 with the Doctor of Public Health degree. He currently is professor of Health and Exercise Science and director of the Human Performance Lab at Appalachian State University in North Carolina. His research focus has been obesity, sports nutrition, aging, exercise immunology, and nutritional assessment from 1985 to the present, with more than 140 peer-reviewed publications in journals and books. He is also the primary author of six books on sports medicine, physical fitness, and nutrition, and a co-author on two others.

Dr. Nieman sits on the editorial boards of eight journals. He also serves as president of the International Society of Exercise and Immunology, is a member the ACSM National Registry Board for the Registered Clinical Exercise Physiologist, and sits on the medical advisory board for the Total Bally Fitness Corporation. Dr. Nieman was an acrobatic gymnast for 10 years, and has run a total of 58 marathons and ultramarathons.

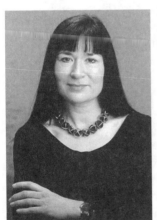

Bente Klarlund Pedersen, MD, Ph.D., graduated from Copenhagen University in 1983 as a medical doctor. She is a specialist in internal medicine and infectious medicine, and works as a clinician in the Department of Infectious Medicine at Rigshospitalet in Copenhagen, Denmark.

Dr. Pedersen's research focus has been exercise and stress immunology, HIV immunology, and aging immunology, with more than 200 peer-reviewed publications in journals and books. She is the author of *Exercise Immunology*, published in 1997 by Springer-Verlag.

Dr. Pedersen is an associate editor of the *Journal of the Danish Medical Association* and a member of the editorial board of the *European Journal of Applied Physiology*. She is president of The Danish Society of Infectious Medicine and past-president of the International Society of Exercise and Immunology.

Contributors

Michael Gleeson, BSc, Ph.D.
Sport and Exercise Sciences
University of Birmingham
Birmingham, England

Peter J. Horvath, Ph.D.
Physical Therapy, Exercise and
 Nutrition Sciences and Physiology
State University of New York at Buffalo
Buffalo, NY

Laurel T. Mackinnon, Ph.D., FACSM, FSMA
Human Movement Studies
The University of Queensland
Brisbane, Australia

David C. Nieman, Dr.PH, FACSM
Health, Leisure, and Exercise Science
Appalachian State University
Boone, NC

Kenneth Ostrowski, Ph.D.
Copenhagen Muscle Research Center
Infectious Disease
Rigshospitalet,
University of Copenhagen, Denmark

Bente K. Pedersen, MD, Ph.D.
Copenhagen Muscle Research Center
Infectious Diseases
Rigshospitalet
University of Copenhagen, Denmark

David R. Pendergast, Ph.D.
Physiology
State University of New York at Buffalo
Buffalo, NY

Edith M. Peters, MSc
Physiology
Faculty of Medicine
University of Natal
Durban, South Africa

Thomas Rohde, Ph.D.
Copenhagen Muscle Research Center
Infectious Diseases
Rigshospitalet
University of Copenhagen, Denmark

David G. Rowbottom, Ph.D.
Human Movement Studies
Queensland University of Technology
Brisbane, Australia

Jaya T. Venkatraman, Ph.D.
Physical Therapy, Exercise and
 Nutrition Sciences
State University of New York at Buffalo
Buffalo, NY

Jeffrey A. Woods, Ph.D.
Kinesiology
University of Illinois
 at Urbana/Champaign
Urbana, IL

Contents

CHAPTER 1

Exercise Immunology: Current Issues

Laurel T. Mackinnon

CONTENTS

1-8493-0741-4/00/$0.00+$.50

1.1. INTRODUCTION

Interest in the effects of physical exertion on the immune system has a long history in many cultures, dating at least as far back as the ancient Greeks. Although papers on this topic appear in the western scientific literature sporadically from the late 19th century, not until the mid-1980s did a field of study that could be defined as exercise immunology first appear.

Current interest in exercise immunology arises from four main directions:[1] First, athletes, coaches and sport physicians have long believed that athletes are susceptible to infectious illness — mainly upper respiratory tract infection (URTI) — during intense training and after major competition. Second, since physical inactivity is now acknowledged as a major risk factor for several lifestyle-associated diseases (e.g., cardiovascular disease), there is interest in whether a lifetime of regular moderate exercise also helps prevent infectious diseases or cancer. Third, there are many potential clinical applications. Exercise is now an integral part of management or rehabilitation for a number of diseases with significant involvement of the immune system, such as cancer, rheumatoid arthritis, and HIV-AIDS, and it is of interest to determine whether exercise influences disease progress and patient prognosis. In addition, attention has focused on whether exercise may reverse or prevent immune suppression associated with, for example, space flight or aging. Finally, the close communication between the neuroendocrine and immune systems implies that activation of the neuroendocrine system (e.g., release of stress hormones that occurs during exercise) has potential to modulate immune function. Indeed, as discussed later in this chapter, much of the acute immune response to exercise can be mechanistically linked to changes in stress hormones.

1.2. OVERVIEW OF THE LITERATURE ON EXERCISE IMMUNOLOGY

The immune response to any stimulus is complex, requiring coordinated action by several types of cells in a tightly regulated sequence. Thus, a physical stress such as exercise may act at any number of points in the complex sequence of events collectively termed the immune response.[1] This point should be kept in mind when reading the literature on exercise immunology, because not all immune parameters respond similarly to the same exercise stress. For example, although exercise causes many profound changes in parameters of immune function, the nature and magnitude of such changes depend on several factors including the immune parameter of interest; type (mode), intensity, and duration of exercise; fitness level or exercise history of the subject; environmental factors such as ambient temperature; and the time course of measurement. In general, the magnitude of change in any immune parameter is a function of exercise dosage (intensity and duration). As discussed later in this chapter and throughout this book, much of the response can be explained by the effects of stress hormones released during exercise.

The exercise immunology literature has focused on resistance to infection as well as key components of immune function, such as leukocytes (immune cells), soluble messenger molecules (e.g., cytokines), soluble factors with effector functions (e.g., immunoglobulin), and other factors that might influence cellular function or release of soluble factors (e.g., glutamine); each of these will be discussed separately below. Responses to acute (single exercise session) as compared with chronic (long-term adaptations), and moderate as compared with intense exercise are also discussed, since these impact on the magnitude and direction of change.

1.2.1 URTI in Athletes

Symptoms of URTI (e.g., runny nose, nasal congestion, sore throat) are often reported by athletes, especially participants in endurance sports requiring high volume training (e.g., distance runners, competitive swimmers, rowers).[2,3] The incidence of URTI appears to be highest after major competition or during high volume training. As many as 50%–70% of such athletes may report symptoms of URTI during the two weeks following major competition (e.g, marathon or ultramarathon running).[4-6] Moreover, URTI incidence is related to training volume in distance runners;[2,6] risk may be elevated by two–four times in the highest compared with lowest volume runners. Short-term intense exercise training is also associated with a high risk of URTI; for example, 42% of competitive swimmers exhibited symptoms of URTI during a 4-week period of intensified training.[7]

In contrast, moderate exercise is not associated with an elevated risk of URTI, and may possibly reduce susceptibility to illness.[8] A 'J-curve' model has been proposed to describe the relationship between exercise volume (intensity and duration combined) and susceptibility to URTI, in which risk of URTI would be reduced by moderate activity but progressively elevated by increasingly intense exercise. While much of the data on URTI in athletes are generally supportive of this model (i.e., that excessive exercise elevates risk of URTI), there are too few data to unequivocally support the notion that moderate exercise lowers risk over the long term. From the public health perspective, the minimum and optimum amounts of exercise to modify risk of URTI or other infectious diseases are currently unknown. At the other end, for the high-performance athlete who must undertake intense exercise on a daily basis, it is of interest to identify ways to minimize adverse effects of exercise on immunity to avoid illness (discussed further below and throughout this book).

1.2.2 Effects of Exercise on Leukocyte (Immune Cell) Number

Leukocytes are a heterogeneous group of immune cells found in several lymphoid tissues and organs, and in the blood and lymph. Table 1.1 presents a summary of the different types of leukocytes and their prevalence in the circulation. Leukocytes display unique cell surface antigens that are used to identify and study the number and function of various subsets; by international agreement, these cell surface proteins are identified by the prefix CD (cluster of differentiation). Leukocytes continually circulate among the blood, lymph, and various lymphoid tissues and organs. Because of obvious limitations in access, research on the human immune response to exercise is restricted to leukocytes obtained from peripheral blood, which may represent only 1%–2% of all immune cells in the body at any given time. Thus, sampling immune cells from human blood may be said to provide a "window" with

Table 1.1 Summary of Immune Cell Subsets and Functions Studied in Exercise Immunology Literature

Cell and Main Identifying CD (where relevant)	Prevalence in Human Peripheral Blood	Major Cell Functions
Polymorphonuclear granulocytes (mainly neutrophils)	70% of leukocytes	Phagocytosis, degradation of damaged tissue
Monocyte (CD14)	10–15% of leukocytes	Phagocytosis, antigen-presentation, cytokine production, cytotoxicity
Lymphocyte	20–25% of leukocytes	Initiate immune response, cytokine production, cytotoxicity, memory
T lymphocyte (CD3)	60–75% of lymphocytes	Immune regulation, cytokine production, immune cell activation, memory
Helper/inflammatory T cell (CD4)	60–70% of T cells	Immune cell activation, antigen recognition, cytokine production
Cytotoxic/suppressor T cell (CD8)	30–40% of T cells	Cytotoxicity
Natural-killer (NK) cell (CD16, 56)	5–20% of lymphocytes	Cytotoxicity, cytokine production
B cell (CD19, 20)	5–15% of lymphocytes	Antibody production, memory

which to view immune events occurring throughout the body. The underlying assumption (which may not always be correct) is that the activity of cells in the blood reflects the activity of cells in the entire body.

1.2.2.1 Acute Exercise Effects

Exercise induces dramatic changes in the number and subset distribution of circulating leukocytes, many of which appear to be mediated by release of stress hormones such as corticosteroids and catecholamines.[1] Circulating leukocyte number could increase up to four times resting levels, and might continue to increase up to several hours after exercise (Figure 1.1). In general, the magnitude of leukocytosis (increase in leukocyte number) is proportional to exercise intensity and duration, although duration is probably more influential. The time course of exercise leukocytosis is complex and may be biphasic, depending on exercise intensity and duration. Leukocyte number may increase during and up to 30 min after brief, intense exercise, return to baseline levels and then increase again 1–3 h post-exercise. Such biphasic response is generally not seen with longer duration (i.e., > 30 min) exercise.

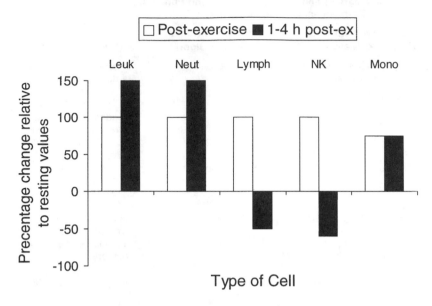

Figure 1.1   Summary of the time course of changes in circulating leukocyte number during
and after intense prolonged exercise. Abbreviations: post-ex = post-exercise recovery period; leuk = total leukocyte count, neut = neutrophil count, lymph = lymphocyte count, NK = natural killer cell count, mono = monocyte count. Values are
expressed relative to resting values; values > 0 reflect increased number and
values < 0 reflect decreased number of cells relative to resting values. (Compiled
from many sources.)

Leukocytosis (and changes in the relative distribution of subsets, see below) is
transitory, returning to baseline levels within several hours after the end of exercise.

The increase in circulating leukocyte number is mirrored by similar changes in
polymorphonuclear granulocyte (primarily neutrophil) counts. Neutrophils are
recruited into the circulation by cortisol released during and after intense exercise,
and cell counts may increase (neutrophilia) to four times resting levels. Neutrophil
number generally returns to baseline levels within 1 h after moderate exercise, but
may remain elevated above resting values for 6 h after intense prolonged exercise
(see Figure 1.1).[1]

Lymphocytosis (increase in lymphocyte concentration) occurs during exercise
(whether brief or intense), but to a lesser extent than changes in neutrophil number.
Various lymphocyte subsets may respond differently to acute exercise, resulting in
changes in the relative proportions of T, B, and NK cells (Figure 1.1). NK cell
number increases the most during and immediately after intense exercise, sometimes
achieving values three times higher than at rest. T cell number increases to a lesser
extent during exercise. Although both CD4 (helper/inflammatory) and CD8 (cyto-
toxic/suppressor) T cell counts increase, the ratio of CD4 to CD8 T cells generally
declines due to relatively larger increases in CD8 than CD4 cell numbers. Exercise
induces little change in B cell numbers, and any change does not persist for long
after the end of exercise. Lymphocytosis also exhibits a biphasic response, although

of a different pattern than for neutrophils. While lymphocyte count increases during and immediately after exercise, values may decline below pre-exercise counts between 1 and 4 hours after intense exercise (Figure 1.1). This biphasic response is reflected in changes in lymphocyte subsets, that is, concentrations of NK, CD4, and CD8 cells all tend to decline below pre-exercise values 1–4 h after intense exercise. Monocyte number increases by about 50% immediately after exercise and may remain elevated for up to 4–6 h post-exercise (Figure 1.1).

Table 1.2 Evidence for Immune Suppression During Intense Exercise Training in Athletes

Immune Parameter*	Major Finding	Key Reference(s)
Leukocyte count*	Progressive decrease toward clinically low levels after 4 wk intense run training	9
Neutrophil activity	Lower resting and post-exercise values in cyclists than in non-athletes	24
	Less increase after exercise in runners during intense training than in moderate training and non-athletes	22
	Progressive decrease as exercise intensity increased during training season in swimmers	28
NK cell number and function*	Declining NK cell number during 10 days' intense run training in military personnel	10
	Progressive decrease in NK cell number over 7 mo training season in swimmers	11
Mucosal IgA	Lower at rest in Nordic skiers than in non-athletes and decrease after races	52
	Progressive decrease over 7-mo training season in swimmers	11
	Lower in overtrained than in well-trained	53
	Acute decrease related to appearance of URTI in hockey and squash athletes	50
	Declines over 7-mo season related to appearance of URTI	11
Serum Ig	Clinically low levels during 7-mo training season in swimmers	11
	Normal specific antibody response to antigenic challenge	46,47
Plasma glutamine	Resting levels lower in overtrained athletes	7,56
	Progressive decrease over 10 days' intense run training in military personnel	57
	Progressive decline over 8 wk intense run training	58

*All data from human peripheral blood except for mucosal IgA measured in saliva.

1.2.2.2 Chronic Training Effects

Exercise-induced changes in circulating leukocyte and subset numbers are transitory, and cell counts usually return to normal levels by 12 to 24 h after exercise.

Thus, providing a blood sample is obtained from an athlete in a truly rested state (i.e., > 24 h after the last exercise session), there appear to be few chronic effects of exercise training on immune-cell number, and clinically normal levels are observed in most athletes. The possible exception is during prolonged periods of very intense training when some athletes may show clinically low cell concentrations[9] or NK cell number may decline.[10,11] For example, progressively declining leukocyte counts (from 5.4 to 4.2 x $10^9 \cdot L^{-1}$), were reported in runners during 4-week intensified training that resulted in symptoms of the overtraining syndrome (stress response to excessive training)(Table 1.2)[9]; the final values were near the low end of the clinically normal range (4-11 x $10^9 \cdot L^{-1}$). In general, however, it does not appear that normal training as performed by most athletes alters circulating immune cell number, although it is not known at present whether cell turnover is altered.

1.2.2.3 Mechanisms Underlying Immune Cell Number Changes

Changes in immune cell numbers and relative proportions of subsets are transitory, and cell number is generally restored to normal values within several hours after exercise. Thus, increases in cell number during and after exercise reflect influx of cells into the circulation, and restoration of normal values after exercise reflects removal of cells from the circulation. During exercise, cells are recruited into the circulation from the "marginated" pools in underperfused areas of the lung[12] and from the spleen.[13] Mechanisms responsible for the increase in cell numbers involve a combination of: (a) increase in cardiac output and pulmonary blood flow;[12] (b) release of catecholamines (primarily lymphocytes and NK cells) and cortisol (primarily neutrophils);[14, 15] (c) hyperthermia, acting through changes in catecholamines;[16] (d) possible sympathetic stimulation of the spleen or other lymphoid tissues to release cells;[13] (e) changes in expression of adhesion molecules;[17] and (f) possible apoptosis (DNA-induced damage leading to cell death) of leukocytes.[18] Some of these issues are discussed further below.

1.2.3 Exercise-Induced Changes in Immune Cell Function

Despite only transient perturbation in immune cell number as a result of exercise, there is evidence that both acute and chronic exercise influence some immune cell functions, such as natural killer (NK) cell cytotoxic activity, neutrophil activation and antibacterial activity, lymphocyte proliferation, and monocyte/macrophage function. As discussed further below, some of these changes in function (e.g., NK cytotoxic activity, lymphocyte proliferation) can be attributed to changes in cell number and/or redistribution, while others occur independently of changes in cell number (e.g., neutrophil activation).

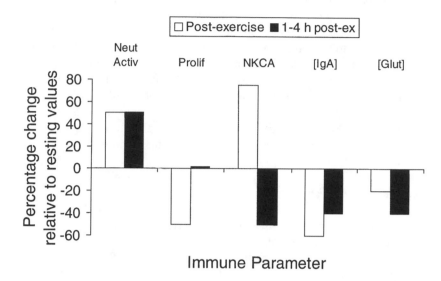

Figure 1.2 Summary of the time course of changes in selected immune parameters during and after intense prolonged exercise. Abbreviations: Neut activ = neutrophil activation; NKCA = natural killer cell cytotoxic activity; [IgA] = salivary IgA concentration; [glut] = plasma glutamine concentration. (Compiled from many sources.)

1.2.3.1 NK Cytotoxic Activity

Much attention has centered on the NK cell response to exercise, since these cells are involved in the early response to viral infection and tumor growth. NK cells also secrete some cytokines, which in turn may influence the activities of other cells. Exercise causes profound changes in both the number of NK cells in the circulation and their cytotoxic (killing) activity. In general, the magnitude and direction of these responses depend on exercise intensity and duration. As discussed above, NK cell number increases up to three times resting levels during and immediately after prolonged intense exercise, but declines below baseline values between 1 and 6 h post-exercise. Thus, NK cells appear to be quickly recruited into the circulation during and leave the circulation rapidly at the end of exercise; such movements may be partially explained by changes in circulating catecholamine levels and adhesion molecule expression.[17] Changes in NK cell number might partially account for changes in NKCA (discussed below).

NK cytotoxic activity (NKCA) increases acutely during exercise in proportion to exercise intensity; NKCA can double after intense prolonged exercise. NKCA returns to resting values soon after brief or moderate exercise,[19,20] but declines and remains below resting levels for up to 6 h after intense prolonged exercise (Figure 1.2).[21] There is much debate about the mechanisms responsible for this delayed decline in NKCA during recovery after exercise, in particular whether it reflects a true suppression of cellular activity or simply the redistribution (hence, change in number) of NK cells in the circulation.[1] Because the NKCA assay uses a mixture of cells (rather than purified NK cells), total NKCA reflects both the killing activity of each cell and the number and relative proportion of NK cells in the blood; each of these can be independently influenced by exercise. Mathematical adjustment of NKCA to account for changes in cell number indicate that NKCA increases during and immediately after exercise because of increased circulating NK cell number. The delayed post-exercise suppression of NKCA is more difficult to explain, and probably reflects a combined effect of several variables including decreasing NK cell number (NK cells exit the circulation), suppression of killing activity by prostaglandins and other substances, and possibly lower sensitivity of NK cells to cytokines. NKCA does not appear to be significantly altered by long-term exercise training, although NK cell number may decline during periods of intense exercise training (Table 1.2).

1.2.3.2 Neutrophil Function

Neutrophil function can be assessed via a variety of *in vitro* assays designed to simulate the complex sequence of events occurring *in vivo* when a neutrophil encounters a pathogenic microorganism such as a bacterium. Briefly, these may be described as migration to sites of tissue injury, phagocytosis (engulfing and destroying) a foreign agent, release of proteolytic enzymes (degranulation), and activation (release of toxic reactive molecules).

Although acute moderate exercise does not appear to alter neutrophil activity, intense exercise stimulates a variety of neutrophil functions, including migration, activation, degranulation, and phagocytosis (Figure 1.2). This stimulation may persist for at least 6 and sometimes up to 24 h after intense prolonged exercise (e.g., 2 h at 75% VO_{2max}).[22-24] Part of the exercise-induced increase in neutrophil activation appears to be due to recruitment into the circulation of younger cells with a higher responsiveness.[24,25] It is thought that activation and/or recruitment of a more active cell occurs in response to skeletal muscle damage, which may elicit release of inflammatory mediators or chemotactic factors that attract neutrophils into the circulation and then to sites of tissue damage. Several studies have reported neutrophil infiltration into tissues such as nasal mucosa,[23] heart and liver,[26] and skeletal muscle[26,27] after intense exercise.

Although acute exercise appears to stimulate neutrophil function, both resting and post-exercise neutrophil function are attenuated in athletes compared with untrained subjects[22,24] or after short-term intense exercise training (Table 1.2).[25] For example, lower neutrophil activation and sensitivity to activating agents were reported in neutrophils obtained both at rest and up to 6 h after exercise in trained cyclists compared with matched non-athletes.[24] Moreover, in distance runners, neutrophil phagocytic activity and activation were lower at rest and 24 h after exercise during intense training than with moderate training or control subjects.[22] In addition, neutrophil activation and sensitivity to activating agents were also reported to decline as training intensity increased during a 12-week period of intense training in competitive swimmers.[28] Taken together, these studies suggest that acute exercise stimulates neutrophil function, but that prolonged periods of intense training are associated with downregulation of neutrophil function. Acute stimulation of neutrophil function is thought to result from a combination of factors including recruitment into the circulation of more-active cells; release of certain cytokines such as IL-1 or TNFα, or hormones such as growth hormone or catecholamines; or tissue-damage-causing release of chemotactic factors. It has been suggested that the apparent downregulation of neutrophil function in athletes may be protective by limiting neutrophil involvement in the inflammatory response initiated by intense daily exercise (discussed further below).

1.2.3.3 Lymphocyte Proliferation

Lymphocytes are activated upon exposure to antigens, after which they enter the cell cycle and proliferate. Lymphocyte proliferation can be measured in an *in vitro* assay in which cells are exposed to particular mitogens (substances that induce mitosis), simulating the *in vivo* response to naturally occurring antigens. Lymphocyte proliferation is sensitive to exercise intensity and duration.[29,30] Brief moderate exercise appears to have little effect on, or may slightly stimulate, lymphocyte proliferation, whereas intense or prolonged exercise suppresses the proliferative response (Figure 1.2).[31,32] Suppression of lymphocyte proliferation may last up to 3 h after intense prolonged exercise, but normal function is usually restored within 2–6 h after exercise.[32]

The cause of suppression of lymphocyte function after intense exercise is not clear at present but is most likely due to a combination of factors including redistribution of lymphocyte subsets[29,30,33] and suppression of lymphocyte activation or proliferation by some as yet unidentified factor. As described above, lymphocyte number declines 1–4 h after intense exercise, and the relative proportion of lymphocyte subsets also changes. Since *in vitro* assays use a given volume of blood or given number of immune cells, any change in cell number or proportion of T (especially CD4 T cells) to other subsets might reduce the number of cells responding to mitogen. Mathematical adjustment of lymphocyte proliferation data to account for changes in cell number suggests that proliferation per cell is unchanged after moderate exercise, but might still be reduced by intense prolonged exercise.[29,34] In a recent study in which proliferative capacity was compared between purified T cells and the usual mixture of different leukocytes obtained after intense interval exercise, suppression was not observed in isolated cells, but was noted in the cell mixtures.[33] Moreover, infusion of epinephrine at physiological concentrations induced suppression of lymphocyte proliferation similar to that observed during exercise, which was attributed to changes in lymphocyte subset distribution.[35] These data suggest that much of the suppression of lymphocyte proliferation immediately post-exercise could be explained by changes in lymphocyte number and subset ratios. On the other hand, a recent study suggests that lymphocyte redistribution cannot fully account for the delayed depressed proliferation observed after exercise, and that, like NKCA, may depend on the time course of blood sampling.[34] For example, when data were not adjusted for changes in cell number, lymphocyte proliferation was suppressed 2 h after 60 min exercise at 75% VO_{2max}. However, adjusting data to account for changing cell number showed suppression of proliferation (expressed per lymphocyte) immediately but not 2 h post-exercise. Moreover, although lymphocyte number and cortisol concentration were influenced by dietary carbohydrate, diet had no effect on lymphocyte proliferation. These data suggest that a complex combination of factors influences lymphocyte proliferative responses to exercise. Exercise training, whether moderate or intense, does not appear to significantly alter lymphocyte proliferation measured at rest or after exercise.[31,36]

1.2.3.4 Monocyte/Macrophage Function

Monocyte and macrophage functions can be altered both acutely and chronically by exercise. These changes may influence other immune functions since monocytes and macrophages are involved in many aspects of immunity including release of cytokines, phagocytosis, antigen-presentation, and tumor cytotoxicity. Cytokines, such as IL-1, IL-6 and TNFα, appearing in blood and urine during recovery after intense exercise may originate from monocytes activated by exercise.[37] Exercise induces expression of adhesion molecules on monocytes, which might stimulate migration of these cells to sites of tissue injury.[17] Enhanced macrophage anti-tumor activity has been reported after both moderate and exhaustive exercise in mice.[38] While most studies suggest activation of some monocyte/macrophage functions by exercise, a recent study suggests that exhaustive exercise may suppress macrophage expression of MHCII, a receptor involved in antigen-presentation by macrophages.[39] Thus, while some monocyte and macrophage functions (e.g., cytotoxicity, adherence) may be stimulated acutely by exercise, there is some evidence of suppression, at least in an animal model, of other aspects of monocyte/macrophage activity (e.g., MHCII expression and possibly antigen-presentation).

1.2.4 Soluble Factors

Soluble factors are found in blood and other body fluids and act as mediators of immune function by activating cells, by mediating communication between different types of cells, by mediating movement of cells throughout the body, by directly killing certain pathogens, or by providing nutrients or substrates required by immune cells. The major soluble factors studied in the exercise immunology literature are cytokines, immunoglobulins, and glutamine. They are discussed separately in the following sections.

1.2.4.1 Cytokines

Cytokines are regulatory molecules involved in communication between immune and other cells. Intense prolonged exercise induces release of several cytokines including those involved in inflammation, such as interleukin-1 (IL-1), IL-6, and tumor necrosis factor-α (TNFα), and in antiviral activity such as interferon-α/β (IFN-α/β).[40,41] In general, cytokines are released only after intense prolonged exercise (e.g., long-distance running) or exercise with a large eccentric bias (forced lengthening of muscle) that induces muscle cell damage.[42–44]

Changes in plasma levels of cytokines are not always observed after exercise despite other evidence of their release (e.g., appearance in urine), possibly because cytokines act locally and are rapidly removed from the circulation. In plasma, IL-6 is the most consistently observed cytokine to increase after exercise. Secretion and degradation of cytokines, as evidenced by elevated urinary levels, may persist for many hours after exercise, and the time course and magnitude of increase may vary between cytokines. For example, in experienced runners, after a 20-km run, a twofold elevation of urinary IL-1 concentration was observed only between 3 and 24 h after exercise, while a threefold increase in urinary IL-6 concentration was noted immediately and up to 5 h after exercise, gradually returning to pre-exercise values by 24 hours after exercise.[41] Although, after exercise, cytokines may be detected in plasma or in urine, the source and significance remains unresolved at present since cytokines can be produced by many different types of cells and not exclusively by leukocytes; this point is discussed further below.

1.2.4.2 Immunoglobulin and Antibody

Immunoglobulin (Ig) is a general term describing a class of glycoproteins produced by mature B lymphocytes that appear in serum and secretions (e.g., saliva, tears) protecting mucosal surfaces. An Ig that reacts with a specific antigen (foreign protein) is termed an antibody. An antibody has several functions, most importantly the binding of antigen on the surface of foreign cells, which in turn stimulates other immune cells to kill the foreign pathogen. Ig exists in five classes with different functions. The exercise literature has focused mainly on IgA in mucosal secretions (e.g., saliva) and IgG in serum. IgA contained in fluids bathing the oral mucosal surfaces is an important early defense against viruses causing URTI.

Acute exercise and moderate exercise training cause little, if any, change in the concentration of total serum Ig, Ig subclasses (e.g., IgG, IgA) or serum antibody titers to specific antigens.[1,45] In contrast, prolonged periods of intense exercise training may cause reduced serum Ig levels; for example, clinically low IgA and IgG levels were observed in resting samples obtained from elite swimmers (Table 1.2).[11] However, despite clinically low serum Ig levels, elite athletes are still capable of mounting a clinically appropriate antibody response to antigenic challenge.[46,47]

While mucosal IgA concentration does not change after moderate exercise, marked declines in salivary IgA and IgM concentration have been reported after intense prolonged or brief interval exercise (Figure 1.2);[11,48,49] values may remain low for at least 1 h after exercise.[49] In athletes, exercise-induced decreases in salivary IgA concentration might predict the appearance of URTI.[50,51] Clinically low or declining IgA concentration has also been observed in athletes during periods of intense training[11,52] or overtraining (Table 1.2).[53] The mechanisms responsible for decreased mucosal IgA concentration after exercise are unknown at present, and may reflect a combined response to psychological and physiological stress and possibly neuroendocrine factors. To date, IgA concentration is the only immune parameter that has been directly linked to susceptibility to URTI in athletes.[50,51]

1.2.4.3 Glutamine, Exercise, and Immune Function

Glutamine is the most abundant amino acid in the body and is required for normal immune-cell function, acting as both a substrate for energy production and a nitrogen source for nucleotide synthesis (and thus lymphocyte proliferation). Plasma glutamine concentration may decline during and for several hours after intense exercise.[54,55] Plasma glutamine levels appear to be lower in overtrained than in well-trained athletes,[7,56] and may progressively decline after 10 days[57] to 8 weeks[58] of intense exercise training (Table1.2). Lymphocyte uptake and oxidation of glutamine are stimulated by exercise,[59] suggesting that plasma levels might decline because of increased removal from the blood by lymphocytes. Because lymphocytes require a constant supply of glutamine, it has been proposed that low plasma glutamine concentrations occurring acutely after intense exercise, or during periods of intense training, might compromise immunity in athletes.[54,55] At present, empirical data supporting this concept are inconsistent. Plasma glutamine concentration was unrelated to the appearance of URTI in swimmers during 4 weeks of intensified training,[7] despite differences in glutamine levels between overtrained and well-trained athletes. In contrast, glutamine supplementation after competitive distance running was associated with lower incidence of URTI.[60] This topic is discussed further below and in a later chapter.

1.3. CURRENT ISSUES IN EXERCISE IMMUNOLOGY

With maturation of the field of exercise immunology over the past several years, research has changed direction from the primarily descriptive studies of the 1980s and early 1990s (which are, of course, necessary in any new field) to focus more on mechanistic issues. This section will briefly discuss some of the current issues and interesting research questions raised by the most recent literature. The final chapter of this book will discuss future directions for research and applications in exercise immunology.

1.3.1 To What Extent Should Exercise Be Modified During URTI?

Because URTI is a fairly frequent illness, and often occurs at inconvenient times (e.g., during competition) in athletes, the question has been raised as to what extent athletes need to restrict their training during and after URTI. Exercise capacity and muscular strength might be temporarily reduced during viral infection eliciting fever,[61,62] suggesting that athletes could be unable to perform at the expected level during febrile illness. Continuing to train intensely through a viral infection has been attributed to the later onset of chronic fatigue syndrome in some athletes.[63] Moreover, there is some concern that viral myocarditis might result from intense exercise during certain viral illnesses (e.g., those caused by coxsackie virus), based on animal models showing increased myocardial damage in animals forced to exercise during coxsackie infection.[64,65] Although viral myocarditis resulting from exercise is rare in humans, physicians treating athletes are concerned that early return to intense training after some types of viral infection could put the athlete at risk of serious complications such as myocarditis. At present, there are no empirically derived guidelines to help physicians decide when an athlete can safely return to training after viral infection

URTI symptoms can be caused by several different viruses, and the cause of any particular viral URTI can vary by season and location. A question often asked by the competitive athlete is to what extent exercise training should be modified during viral URTI. In a recent study, subjects were exposed to a novel rhinovirus (a class of virus causing about 40% of URTI in North America) and then half the subjects exercised moderately (40 min at 70% of heart rate reserve on alternate days for 10 days).[66] Severity and duration of symptoms were not significantly different between exercised and rested subjects, suggesting that moderate exercise does not influence severity of viral infection. It was noted, however, that these results may not necessarily be applicable to more-intense exercise or to URTI caused by other viruses. Further work is needed to determine whether severity of illness is influenced by more-intense exercise, and whether this response differs between viral agents.

1.3.2 Does Downregulation of Immune Function in Athletes Serve a Useful Purpose?

Certain aspects of nonspecific immunity, in particular neutrophil function, appear to be downregulated during prolonged periods of intense, but not moderate, exercise training in athletes.[22,28,67] Since neutrophils are important in the early defense against many pathogens, it is possible that such suppression adversely influences immune function in athletes. Alternatively, neutrophils are also inflammatory cells, migrating to injured tissue sites (such as damaged skeletal muscle) and secreting toxic factors involved in proteolysis and cellular damage (such as reactive oxygen and nitrogen species). Intense exercise has been shown to induce infiltration of neutrophils into many tissues such as cardiac and skeletal muscle[26] and nasal mucosa,[23] where they may initiate inflammatory processes. Thus, downregulation of neutrophil function in athletes might be protective by limiting chronic inflammation resulting from intense daily exercise. If so, this would imply that slightly suppressed immune function may be a necessary compromise between the processes of inflammation and immune responsiveness.

1.3.3 Can Nutritional Supplements Beneficially Alter the Immune Response to Exercise?

Interest in this question arises from two directions: from the practical viewpoint as to whether athletes can use legal nutritional supplements to prevent immune suppression resulting from intense prolonged exercise, and on the other hand, an experimental focus that uses nutritional manipulation to help identify responsible mechanisms underlying the immune response to exercise. Of course, these two views are not mutually exclusive.

Athletes regularly consume various types of dietary supplements in the belief that these enhance performance or stimulate immune function. As will be discussed throughout this book, there is both theoretical and empirical evidence to support an interaction between nutritional factors and the immune response to exercise. Dietary carbohydrate (CHO) supplementation before and/or during exercise has recently been shown to modulate several aspects of the immune response to intense exercise.

For example, consumption of a 6% CHO "sports drink" during 1–2 h exercise (70-75% VO_{2max}) attenuated the increases in circulating IL-6 concentration and neutrophil and NK cell numbers during exercise, and decline in lymphocyte number and plasma glutamine concentration after exercise.[68–70] The mechanisms underlying these effects are thought to relate to maintenance of plasma glucose concentration and suppression of cortisol release.[69,70] While these studies strongly support the notion that release of immunomodulating hormones such as cortisol underlie many of the immune responses to intense exercise, it is not clear whether CHO supplementation offers useful applications by counteracting adverse effects of intense prolonged exercise on immune function in athletes.

Glutamine and vitamin C are other supplements that have attracted considerable interest from the sports community in the quest to identify supplements that might reduce the risk of URTI or overtraining. The incidence of symptoms of URTI during the two weeks following an ultramarathon was reduced by more than 50% in runners who consumed a vitamin C supplement (600 mg.d[-1]) for three weeks before the race compared with runners consuming a placebo; no effect of vitamin C on URTI incidence was observed in non-athletes, suggesting an effect of vitamin C only when coupled with physical stress.[4,5] Similarly, glutamine supplementation (5 g.d[-1]) has been reported to reduce the incidence of self-reported URTI in the two weeks after competition in distance runners.[60] At present, these remain intriguing observations awaiting further study to determine the extent of, and mechanisms responsible for, this apparent protection against URTI in endurance athletes.

1.3.4 Is Exercise a Useful Countermeasure During Immunosuppressive Events?

It is widely believed (although with little supporting empirical evidence) that moderate exercise has long-term benefits in preventing infectious disease or stimulating immune function. While there may be few measurable effects on healthy populations, it is still possible that moderate exercise may beneficially augment, or at least attenuate a decline in, immune function during times of immunosuppression.

The aging process is associated with progressive declines in immune parameters such as lymphocyte responsiveness. Given the increasing proportion of older individuals in most developed countries, it is of interest to determine whether a lifetime of moderate physical activity, as recommended for general good health, also helps to counteract this apparently inevitable decline in immune function. There is, at present, relatively little known about the long-term adaptations of the immune system to moderate exercise training in the elderly. The possible use of exercise as a countermeasure has applications to other immunosuppressive conditions, such as HIV-infection/AIDS or spaceflight. Spaceflight is associated with general immune suppression secondary to endocrine and blood-volume changes.[71] Compromised immune function may have serious implications during the long-term spaceflight currently planned for a return to the moon, occupation of space stations and perhaps human missions to Mars. Exercise training before and during spaceflight has been suggested as a possible "countermeasure" to prevent or limit adverse effects on immune function.[72] Similarly, regularly exercise also has potential to beneficially affect immune status and functional capacity in HIV-infected patients.[73-75] For example, resistance training may counteract the muscle wasting that often occurs in HIV infection; recent studies show increases in total and lean body mass in HIV-positive men after 12 weeks of resistance training.[74,75]

1.3.5 Are Exercise-Induced Changes in Immune Function Protective Against Cancer?

Human epidemiological data indicate that physical activity is protective against certain forms of cancer, in particular bowel, breast, and some reproductive-system cancers. Experimental data using animal models also support a protective role for exercise, and implicate favorable changes in immune cell function resulting from exercise. For example, recent studies show a relationship between clearance from the lungs of radiolabeled tumor cells and increased NKCA in spleen cells.[76] Tumor retention was also lower in exercise-trained than in sedentary mice, although the degree of protection varied with tumor type.[77] While increases in NK cell cytotoxic activity might partially explain the protective effect of exercise, it appears that this effect varies by type of tumor, and that there may be other innate immune mechanisms involved.[77]

1.3.6 What Mediates Communication Between Skeletal Muscle and the Immune System?

The immune-system response to exercise depends on exercise mode, intensity, and duration; certain stress hormones (e.g., epinephrine, cortisol) have been implicated as mediators of such exercise-induced changes. However, stress hormones cannot completely explain all aspects of immune changes after exercise, and it appears that there is some type of direct communication between metabolic and/or structural events occurring in skeletal muscle and immune cells. For example, eccentric exercise (downhill running) causes larger perturbations of circulating immune cell numbers than concentric exercise (level running) of similar metabolic cost.[78] Two mechanisms involved in such communication may be cytokines released within or localized to skeletal muscle during and after exercise (discussed above), or altered expression of adhesion molecules influencing trafficking of immune cells throughout the body. Adhesion molecules are cell-surface molecules that mediate binding between different types of cells or between a cell and extracellular matrix proteins. Adhesion molecules mediate leukocyte movement throughout the body and especially from the circulation to sites of tissue damage or inflammation. Expression of adhesion molecules is stimulated by a variety of factors including infection, inflammation, cytokines, and exercise. It has been proposed that movement of cells into and out of the circulation during and after exercise may be explained by changes in surface expression of adhesion molecules.[17] Since some pathogenic microorganisms gain entry to cells via adhesion molecules, exercise-induced changes in adhesion molecule expression may have implications for resistance to infectious agents after exercise.

1.3.7 What is the Source of Cytokines Released During Exercise?

Cytokines appear to be released during and after intense prolonged exercise, especially when an eccentric component is present, as evidenced by the presence of cytokines in plasma and urine. The source of these cytokines has not yet been clearly identified. While circulating leukocytes, in particular monocytes, seem a likely source, there is evidence to suggest other sources as well, perhaps even skeletal muscle. IL-1 has been localized to skeletal muscle damaged by eccentric exercise and in proportion to neutrophil accumulation within the muscle.[27] Exercise does not appear to alter cytokine gene expression in peripheral blood immune cells, suggesting that either cytokines are produced by other cells or that exercise influences post-transcriptional processes in leukocytes.[79]

It has been suggested that pro-inflammatory cytokines such as IL-6 are released in response to skeletal muscle cell damage, since plasma levels are higher after eccentric than concentric exercise.[42] In contrast, however, a recent report from the same laboratory suggested that the concentration of IL-6 released after eccentric exercise was unrelated to muscle proteolysis since supplementation with branch-chain amino acids attenuated markers of muscle cell damage (e.g., creatine kinase and amino acid levels in blood), yet did not attenuate IL-6 release.[44] A recent study from the same laboratory using reverse transcriptase polymerase chain reaction (RT-PCR) techniques to identify IL-6 mRNA suggests that IL-6 may be produced within damaged skeletal muscle following prolonged exercise.[43] While IL-6 mRNA was not expressed in muscle biopsies obtained at rest, IL-6 mRNA expression was noted in biopsies obtained immediately and 2 h after marathon running (3 h) in five of eight subjects. mRNA for IL-6 was not detectable at any time in mononuclear cells, indicating that these cells were not the source of this cytokine.

It was noted that, while IL-6 could be produced by activated monocytes and neutrophils, IL-6 mRNA appeared in skeletal muscle immediately after exercise, before these cells accumulate in muscle. Further studies are needed to confirm whether IL-6 is produced by skeletal muscle cells, whether other cytokines are also produced, and to what extent these cytokines are involved in inflammation and repair of damaged muscle.

1.3.8 Does Exercise-Induced DNA Damage in Lymphocytes Alter Immune Function?

Recent studies show evidence of DNA damage and apoptosis in lymphocytes immediately and up to 48 h after intense exercise; such damage may be cumulative, (i.e., it increases with subsequent bouts of intense exercise).[18] A process of programmed cell "suicide" that begins with DNA damage and quickly proceeds to cell death within minutes, apoptosis is considered to play an important role in maintaining a competent immune system by removing activated lymphocytes once their useful effector functions have been achieved. Increased expression of activation markers (e.g., CD 25, CD122, CD45RA/RO) on lymphocytes, suggesting lymphocyte activation, have been observed during or after exercise.[80] It has been suggested that apoptosis may contribute to the decline in circulating lymphocyte number and proliferation 1–4 h after intense exercise,[18] although it is difficult to reconcile evidence of continued apoptosis despite normal cell number and function 24 h post-exercise. It is currently unknown whether such DNA damage and signs of apoptosis lead to cell death in a significant number of lymphocytes and if so, whether particular subsets of lymphocytes are susceptible and whether apoptosis contributes to alteration in immune function as a result of intense exercise.

1.4. CONCLUSIONS

Exercise alters many aspects of immune function, stimulating some immune parameters while suppressing others. In general, there is a dose-response relationship between exercise amount (duration and/or intensity) and specific immune responses. The significance of these changes to long-term health are unclear at present, but there are many potential applications: understanding why endurance athletes are susceptible to upper respiratory tract infection during intense training and finding ways to lessen the risk of illness; explaining how physical activity protects against cancer, and then identifying the optimal amount of exercise to afford protection; providing a scientific basis for exercise prescription guidelines for individuals in immunocompromised states (e.g., aging, spaceflight, HIV infection); and in further understanding the complexities of immune-system regulation.

REFERENCES

1. Mackinnon, L.T., *Advances in Exercise Immunology*, Human Kinetics Publishing, Champaign, IL,1999.
2. Heath, G.W., Macera, C.A., and Nieman, D.C., Exercise and upper respiratory tract infections: Is there a relationship? *Sports Med.,* 14, 353-365, 1992.
3. Nieman, D.C, and Nehlsen-Cannarella, S.L., Exercise and infection. In *Exercise and Disease*, Ed. R.R. Watson, M. Eisinger. CRC, Boca Raton, pp 122-148, 1992.
4. Peters, E.M, and Bateman, E.D., Ultramarathon running and upper respiratory tract infections. *S. Afr. Med. J.*, 64, 582-584, 1983.
5. Peters, E.M., Goetzsche, J.M., Grobbelaar, B., and Noakes, T.D., Vitamin C supplementation reduces the incidence of postrace symptoms of upper respiratory tract infection in ultramarathon runners. *Am. J. Clin. Nutr.,* 57, 170-174, 1993.
6. Nieman, D.C., Johanssen, L.M., Lee, J.W., and Arabatzis, K., Infectious episodes in runners before and after the Los Angeles Marathon. *J. Sports Med. Physical Fitness,* 30, 316-328, 1990.
7. Mackinnon, L.T. and Hooper, S.L., Plasma glutamine concentration and upper respiratory tract infection during overtraining in elite swimmers. *Med. Sci. Sports Exerc.,* 28, 285-290, 1996.
8. Nieman, D.C., Nehlsen-Cannarella, S.L., Henson, D.A., Koch, A.J., Butterworth, D.E., Fagoaga, O.R., and Uttre, A., Immune response to exercise training and/or energy restriction in obese women. *Med. Sci. Sports Exerc.*, 30, 679-686, 1998.

9. Lehmann, M. Mann, H., Gastmann, U., Keul, J., Vtter, D., Steinacker, J.M., and Haussinger, D., Unaccustomed high-mileage vs intensity-training-related changes in performance and serum amino acid levels. *Int. J. Sports Med.*, 17, 187-192, 1996.

10. Fry, R.W., Grove, J.R., Morton, A.R., Zeroni, P.M., Gaudieri, S., and Keast, D., Psychological and immunological correlates of acute overtraining. *Br. J. Sports Med.*, 28, 241-246, 1994.

11. Gleeson M., McDonald, W.A., Cripps, A.W., Pyne, D.B., Clancy, R.L., and Fricker, P.A., The effect on immunity of long term intensive training in elite swimmers. *Clin. Exp. Immunol.*, 102, 210-216, 1995.

12. Fairbarn, M.S., Blackie, S.P., Rardy, R.L., and Hogg, J.C., Comparison of effects of exercise and hyperventilation on leukocyte kinetics in humans. *J. Appl. Physiol.*, 75, 2425-2428, 1993.

13. Nielsen, H.B., Secher, N.H., Kristensen, J.H., Christensen, N.J., Espersen, K., and Pedersen, B.K., Splenectomy impairs lymphocytosis during maximal exercise. *Am. J. Physiol.*, 272 (*Regulatory Integrative Comp. Physiol.* 41), R1847-1852, 1997.

14. Kappel, M., Stadeager, C., Tvede, N., Galbo, H., and Pedersen, B.K., Effects of *in vivo* hyperthermia on natural killer cell activity, *in vitro* proliferative responses and blood mononuclear cell subpopulations. *Clin. Exp. Immunol.*, 84, 175-180, 1991.

15. Nieman, D.C., Immune response to heavy exertion. *J. Appl. Physiol.*, 82, 1385-1394, 1997.

16. Kappel, M. Diamant, J.O.L., Hansen, M.B., Klokker, M., and Pedersen, B.K., Effects of *in vitro* hyperthermia on the proliferative response of blood mononuclear cell subsets, and detection of interleukins 1 and 6, tumour necrosis factor-alpha and interferon-gamma. *Immunol.*, 73, 304-308, 1991.

17. Gabriel, H. and Kindermann, W., Adhesion molecules during immune response to exercise. *Can. J. Physiol. Pharmacol.*, 76, 1-12, 1998.

18. Mars, M., Govender, A., Weston, A., Naicker, V., and Chuturgoon, A., High intensity exercise: a cause of lymphocyte apoptosis?, *Biochem. Biophys. Res. Comm.*, 249, 366-370, 1998.

19. Nielsen, H.B., Secher, H.H., Christensen, N.J., and Pedersen, B.K., Lympocytes and NK cell activity during repeated bouts of maximal exercise. *Am. J. Physiol.* 271 (*Regulatory Integrative Comp. Phsyiol.*, 40), R222-R227, 1996.

20. Nieman, D.C., Miller, A.R., Henson, D.A., Warren, B.J., Gusewitch, G., Johnson, R.L., Davis, J.M., Butterworth, D.E., and Nehlsen-Cannarella, S.L., Effects of high- vs moderate-intensity exercise on natural killer activity. *Med. Sci. Sports Exerc.*, 25, 1126-1134, 1993.

21. Nieman, D.C., Brendle, D., Henson, D.A., Suttles, J., Cook, V.D., Warren, B.J., Butterworth, D.E., Fagoaga, O.R., and Nehlsen-Cannarella, S.L., Immune function in athletes vs nonathletes. *Int. J. Sports Med.*, 16, 329-333, 1995.

22. Hack, B., Strobel, G., Weiss, M., and Weicker, H., PMN cell counts and phagocytic activity of highly trained athletes depend on training period. *J. Appl. Physiol.*, 77, 1731-1735, 1994.

23. Muns, G., Rubinstein, I., and Singer, P., Neutrophil chemotactic activity is increased in nasal secretions of long-distance runners. *Int. J. Sports Med.*, 17, 56-59, 1996.

24. Smith, J.A., Telford, R.D., Mason, I.B., and Weidemann, M.J., Exercise, training and neutrophil microbicidal activity. *Int. J. Sports Med.*, 11, 179-187, 1990.

25. Suzuki, K., Naganuman, S., Totsuka, M., Suzuki, K.-J., Mochizuki, M., Shiraishi, M., Nakaji, S., and Sugawara, K., Effects of exhaustive endurance exercise and its one-week daily repetition on neutrophil count and functional status in untrained men. *Int. J. Sports Med.*, 17, 205-212, 1996.

26. Belcastro, A.N., Arthur, G.D., Albisser, R.A., and Raj, D.A., Heart, liver, and skeletal muscle myeloperoxidase activity during exercise. *J. Appl. Physiol.*, 80, 1331-1335, 1996.

27. Fielding, R.A., Manfredi, T.J., Ding, W., Fiatarone, M.A., Evans, W.J., and Cannon, J.G., Acute phase response in exercise III. Neutrophil and IL-1αβ accumulation in skeletal muscle. *Am. J. Physiol.* (*Regulatory Integrative Comp. Physiol.*, 34), R166-R172, 1993.

28. Pyne, D.B., Baker, M.S., Fricker, P.A., McDonald, W.A., Telford, R.D., and Weidemann, M.J., Effects of an intensive 12-wk training program by elite swimmers on neutrophil oxidative activity. *Med. Sci. Sports Exerc.*, 27, 536-542, 1995.

29. Nieman, D.C., Miller, A.R., Henson, D.A., Warren, G., Johnson, R.L., Davis, J.M., Butterworth, D.E., Herring, J.L., and Nehlsen-Cannarella, S.L., Effect of high- vs moderate-intensity exercise on lymphocyte subpopulations and proliferative response. *Int. J. Sports Med.*, 15, 199-206, 1994.

30. Tvede, N., Kappel, M., Halkjaer-Kristensen, J., Galbo, H., and Pedersen, B.K., The effect of light, moderate and severe bicycle exercise on lymphocyte subsets, natural and lymphokine activated killer cells, lymphocyte proliferative response and interleukin-2 production. *Int. J. Sports Med.*, 14, 275, 282, 1993.

31. Mitchell, J.B., Paquet, A.J., Pizza, F.X., Starling, R.D., Holtz, R.W., and Grandjean, P.W., The effect of moderate aerobic training on lymphocyte proliferation. *Int. J. Sports Med.*, 17, 384-389, 1996.

32. Nieman, D.C., Simandle, S., Henson, D.A., Warren, B.J., Suttles, J., Davis, J.M., Buckely, K.S., Ahle, J.C.,Butterworth, D.E., Fagoaga, O.R., and Nehlsen-Cannarella, S.L., Lymphocyte proliferative response to 2.5 hours of running. *Int. J. Sports Med.*, 16, 404-408, 1995.

33. Hinton, J.R., Rowbottom. D.G., Keast, D., and Morton, A.R., Acute intensive interval training and *in vitro* T-lymphocyte function. *Int. J. Sports Med.*, 18, 132-137, 1997.

34. Mitchell, J.B., Pizza, F.X., Paquet, A., Davis, B.J., Forrest, M.B., and Braun, W.A., Influence of carbohydrate status on immune responses before and after endurance exercise. *J. Appl. Physiol.*, 84, 1917-1925, 1998.

35. Tvede, N.M., Kappel, M., Klarlund, K., Duhn, S., Halkjaer-Kristensen, J., Kjaer, M., Galbo, H., and Pedersen, B.K., Evidence that the effect of bicycle exercise on blood mononuclear cell proliferative responses and subsets is mediated by epinephrine. *Int. J. Sports Med.*, 15, 100-104, 1994.

36. Verde, T.J., Thomas, S.G., and Shephard, R.J., Potential markers of heavy training in highly trained distance runners. *Br. J. Sports Med.*, 26, 167-175, 1992.

37. Woods, J.A. and Davis, J.M., Exercise, monocyte-macrophage function and cancer. *Med. Sci. Sports Exerc.*, 26, 147-157, 1994.

38. Woods, J.A., Davis, J.M., Mayer, E.P., Ghaffar, A., and Pate, R.R., Effects of exercise on macrophage activation for antitumor cytotoxicity. *J. Appl. Physiol.*, 76, 2177-2185, 1994.

39. Woods, J.A., Ceddia, M.A., Kozak, C., and Wolters, B.W., Effects of exercise on the macrophage MHCII response to inflammation. *Int. J. Sports Med.*, 18, 483-488, 1997.

40. Davis, J.M., Weaver, J.A., Kohut, M.L., Colbert, L.H., Ghaffar, A., and Mayer, E.P., Immune system activation and fatigue during treadmill running: role of interferon. *Med. Sci. Sports Exerc.*, 30, 863-868, 1998.

41. Sprenger, H., Jacobs, C. Nain, M., Gressner, A.M., Prinz, H., Wesemann, W., and Gemsa, D., Enhanced release of cytokines, interleukin-2 receptors, and neopterin after long-distance running. *Clin.. Immunol.. Immunopath.*, 53, 188-195, 1992.

42. Bruunsgaard, H., Galbo, H., Halkjaer-Kristensen, J., Johansen, T.L., MacLean, D.A., and Pedersen, B.K., Exercise-induced increase in serum interleukin-6 in humans is related to muscle damage. *J. Physiol.*, 499, 833-841, 1997.

43. Ostrowski, K., Rohde, T., Zacho, M., Asp, S., and Pedersen, B.K., Evidence that interleukin-6 is produced in human skeletal muscle during prolonged running. *J. Physiol.*, 508, 949-953, 1998.

44. 'Rohde, T., MacLean, D.A., Richter, E.A., Kiens, B., and Pedersen, B.K., Prolonged submaximal eccentric exercise is associated with increased levels of plasma IL-6. *Am. J. Physiol.*, 273 (*Endocrinol. Metab.* 36), E85-E91, 1997.

45. Mackinnon, L.T., Exercise, immunoglobulin and antibody. *Exerc. Immunol., Rev.* 2, 1-32, 1996.

46. Bruunsgaard, H., Hartkopp, A., Mohr, T., Konradsen, H., Heron, I., Mordhorst, C. H., and Pedersen, B.K., *In vivo* cell-mediated immunity and vaccination response following prolonged intense exercise. *Med. Sci. Sports Exerc.*, 29, 1176-1181, 1997.

47. Gleeson, M., Pyne, D.B., McDonald, W.A., Clancy, R.L., Cripps, A.W., Horn, P.L., and Fricker, P.A., Pneumococcal antibody response in elite swimmers. *Clin. Exp. Immunol.*, 105, 238-244, 1996.

48. Mackinnon, L.T. and Jenkins, D.G., Decreased salivary IgA after intense interval exercise before and after training. *Med. Sci. Sports Exerc.*, 25, 678-683, 1993.

49. Mackinnon, L.T., Chick, T.W., van As, A., and Tomasi, T.B., Decreased secretory immunoglobulins following intense endurance exercise. *Sports Training Med. Rehab.*, 1, 209-218, 1989.

50. Mackinnon, L.T., Ginn, E., and Seymour, G.J., Temporal relationship between exercise-induced decreases in salivary IgA and subsequent appearance of upper respiratory tract infection in elite athletes. *Aust. J. Sci. Med. Sports*, 25, 94-99, 1993.

51. Gleeson, M., McDonald, W.A., Pyne, D.B., Cripps, A.W., Francis, J.L., Fricker, P.A., and Clancy, R.L., Salivary IgA levels and infection risk in elite swimmers. *Med. Sci. Sports Exerc.*, 31, 67-73, 1999.

52. Tomasi, T.B., Trudeau, F.B., Czerwinski, D., and Erredge, S., Immune parametersin athletes before and after strenuous exercise. *J. Clin. Immunol.*, 2, 173-179, 1982.

53. Mackinnon, L.T. and Hooper, S.L., Mucosal (Secretory) immune system responses to exercise of varying intensity and during overtraining. *Int. J. Sports Med.*, 15, S179-S183, 1994.

54. Rowbottom, D.G., Keast, D., and Morton, A.R., The emerging role of glutamine as an indicator of exercise stress and overtraining. *Sports Med.*, 21, 80-97, 1996.

55. Walsh, N.P., Blannin, A.K., Robson, P.J., and Gleeson, M., Glutamine, exercise and immune function: links and possible mechanisms. *Sports Med.*, 26, 177-191, 1998.

56. Rowbottom D.G., Keast, D., Goodman, C. and Morton, A.R., The haematological, biochemical and immunological profile of athletes suffering from the overtraining syndrome. *Europ. J. Appl. Physiol.*, 70, 502-509, 1995.

57. Keast, D., Arstein, D., Harper, W., Fry, R.W., and Morton, A.R., Depression of plasma glutamine concentration after exercise stress and its possible influence on the immune system. *Med. J. Aust.*, 162, 15-18, 1995.

58. Hack, V., Weiss, C., Friedmann, B., Suttner, S., Schykowski, M., Erbe, N., Benner, A., Bartsch, P., and Droge, W., Decreased plasma glutamine level and CD4+ T cell number in response to 8 wk of anaerobic training. *Am. J. Physiol.*, 272 (*Endocrinol. Metab.* 35), E788-E795, 1997.

59. Frisina, J.P., Gaudieri, S., Cable, T., Keast, D., and Palmer, T. N., Effect of acute exercise on lymphocyte subsets and metabolic activity. *Int. J. Sports Med.*, 15, 36-41, 1994.

60. Castell, L.M. and Newsholme, E.A., The effects of oral glutamine supplementation on athletes are prolonged, exhaustive exercise. *Nutrition*, 13, 738-742, 1997.
61. Daniels, W.L., Sharp, D.S., Wright, J.E., Vogel, J.A., Friman, G., Beisel, W.R., and Knapik, J.J., Effects of virus infection on physical performance in man. *Military Med.*, 150, 1-8, 1985.
62. Friman, G., Wright, J.E., Ilback, N.-G., Beisel, W.R., White, J.E., Sharp, D.S., Stephen, E.L., and Daniels, W.L., Does fever of myalgia indicate reduced physical performance capacity in viral infections? *Acta Med. Scand.*, 217, 353-361, 1985.
63. Parker, S., Brukner, P.D., and Rosier, M., Chronic fatigue syndrome and the athlete. *Sports Med., Training, Rehab.*, 6, 269-278, 1996.
64. Ilback, N.-G., Fohlman, J., and Friman, G., Exercise in coxsackie B3 myocarditis: effects on heart lymphocyte subpopulations and the inflammatory reaction. *Am. Heart J.*, 117, 1298-1302, 1989.
65. Kiel, R.J., Smith, F.F., Chason, J., Khatib, R., and Reyes, M.P., Coxsackie B3 myocarditis in C3H/HeJ mice: description of an inbred model and the effect of exercise on virulence. *Europ. J. Epidemiol.*, 5, 348-350, 1989.
66. Weidner, T.G., Cranston, T., Schurr, T., and Kaminsky, L.A., The effect of exercise training on the severity and duration of a viral upper respiratory illness. *Med. Sci. Sports Exerc.*, 30, 1578-1583, 1998.
67. Smith, J.A., Neutrophils, host defense, and inflammation: a double-edged sword. *J. Leukocyte Biol.*, 56, 672-686, 1994.
68. Gleeson, M., Blannin, A.K., Walsh, N.P., Bishop, N.C., and Clark, A.M., Effect of low- and high-carbohydrate diets on the plasma glutamine and circulating leukocyte response to exercise. *Int. J. Sports Nutr.*, 8, 49-59, 1998.
69. Nieman, D.C., Henson, D.A., Garner, E.B., Butterworth, D.E., Warren, B.J., Utter, A., Davis, J.M., Fagoaga, O.R., and Nehlsen-Cannarella, S.L., Carbohydrate affects natural killer cell redistribution but not activity after running. *Med. Sci. Sports Exerc.*, 29,1318-1324, 1997.
70. Nieman, D.C., Nehlsen-Cannarella, S.L., Fagoaga, O. R., Henson, D.A., Utter, A., Davis, J.M., Williams, F., and Butterworth, D.E., Influence of mode and carbohydrate on the cytokine response to heavy exertion. *Med. Sci. Sports Exerc.*, 30, 671-678, 1998.
71. Levine, D.S. and Greenleaf, J.E., Immunosuppression during spaceflight deconditioning. *Aviation, Space, Environ. Med.*, 69, 172-177, 1998.
72. Tipton, C.M., Greenleaf, J.E., and Jackson, C.G.R., Neuroendocrine and immune system responses with spaceflight. *Med. Sci. Sports Exerc.*, 28, 988-998, 1996.
73. Rigsby, L., Dishman, R.,K., Jackson, K.W., Maclean, G.S., and Raven, P.B., Effects of exercise training on men seropositive for the human immunodeficiency virus-1. *Med. Sci. Sports Exerc.*, 24, 6-12, 1992.
74. Spence, D.W., Galatino, M.L.A., Mossberg, K.A., and Zimmermann, S.O., Progressive resistance exercise: effect on muscle function and anthropometry of a select AIDS population. *Arch. Physical Med. Rehab.*, 71, 644-648, 1990.
75. Wagner, G., Rabkin, J., and Rabkin, R., Exercise as a mediator of psychological and nutritional effects of testosterone therapy in HIV+ men. *Med. Sci. Sports Exerc.*, 30, 811-817, 1998.
76. MacNeil, B. and Hoffman-Goetz, L., Chronic exercise enhances *in vivo* and *in vitro* cytotoxic mechanisms of natural immunity in mice. *J. Appl. Physiol.*, 74, 388-395, 1993.
77. Jadeski, L. and Hoffman-Goetz, L., Exercise and *in vivo* natural cytotoxicity against tumour cells of varying metastatic capacity. *Clin. Exp. Metastasis,* 14, 138-144, 1996.

78. Pizza, F.X., Mitchell, J.B., Davis, B.H., Starling, R.D., Holtz, R.W., and Bigelow, N., Exercise-induced muscle damage: effect on circulating leukocyte and lymphocyte subsets. *Med. Sci. Sports Exerc.*, 27, 363-370, 1995.
79. Ullum, H., Martin, P., Diamant, M., Palmo, J., Halkjaer-Kristensen, J., and Pedersen, B.K., Bicycle exercise enhances plasma IL-6 but does not change IL-1α, IL-1β, or TNF-α pre-mRNA in BMNC. *J. Appl. Physiol.*, 77, 93-97, 1994.
80. Gabriel, H., Schmitt, B., Urhausen, A., and Kindermann, W., Increased CD45RA+CD45RO⁻ cells indicate activated T cells after endurance exercise. *Med. Sci. Sports Exerc.*, 25, 1352-1357, 1993.

CHAPTER 2

Carbohydrates and the Immune Response to Prolonged Exertion

David C. Nieman

CONTENTS

2.1 INTRODUCTION

As summarized in Figure 2.1, publications on the topic of exercise immunology date from late in the 19th century. It was not until the mid-1980s, however, that a significant number of investigators worldwide devoted their resources to this area of research endeavor. From 1900 to 1999, just under 1,200 papers on exercise immunology were published, with 78% of these appearing in the 1990s.[1]

Exercise immunology is based on several lines of evidence:[2–4]

1-8493-0741-4/00/$0.00+$.50
© 2000 by CRC Press LLC

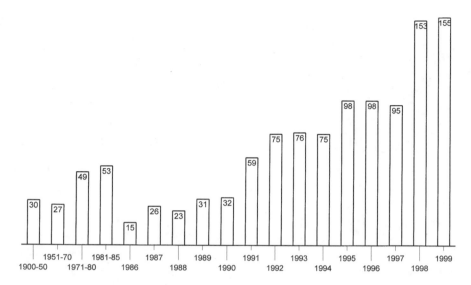

Figure 2.1   There have been nearly 1,200 exercise immunology publications during the 1900s, with 78% of these published within the 1990s.

- Anecdotal data from athletes
- Survey data taken from groups of athletes
- Epidemiologic data
- Studies using animal models
- Cross-sectional studies comparing athletes and nonathletes
- Human studies on the acute and chronic influence of exercise on immune function

In this chapter, emphasis will be placed on exercise immunology studies with human athletes (cross-sectional comparisons with nonathletes, and acute and chronic changes in immunity with exercise), and the role of carbohydrate supplementation as a potential nutritional countermeasure to exercise-induced alterations in immune function.

2.2 INFECTION RATES AND IMMUNITY
IN ENDURANCE ATHLETES

A common perception among elite athletes and their coaches is that prolonged and intense exertion lowers resistance to upper respiratory tract infection (URTI).[2-4] In a 1996 survey conducted by the Gatorade Sports Science Institute, 89% of 2,700 high school and college coaches and athletic trainers checked "yes" to the question, "Do you believe overtraining can compromise the immune system and make athletes sick?" (personal communication, Gatorade Sports Science Institute, Barrington, IL). Several studies using epidemiological designs have verified that URTI risk is elevated during periods of heavy training and in the 1–2 week period following participation in competitive endurance races.[5-8] It should be emphasized, however, that the majority of endurance athletes do not experience URTI after competitive race events. For example, only one in seven marathon runners reported an episode of URTI following the March, 1987, Los Angeles Marathon.[5] URTI rates in marathon runners are even lower during the summer than in winter. In a study of 170 experienced marathon runners, only 3% reported an URTI during the week after a July marathon race event (unpublished data, author, 1993).

A more important survey finding is the common belief among fitness enthusiasts that regular exercise confers resistance against infection. In the same survey noted in the previous paragraph, of 170 non-elite marathon runners (personal best time, an average of 3 h 25 min) who had been training for and participating in marathons for an average of 12 years, 90% reported that they definitely or mostly agreed with the statement that they "rarely get sick." Three randomized exercise training studies have demonstrated that near daily exercise by previously sedentary women for 12–15 weeks is associated with a significant reduction in URTI.[9-11]

The relationship between exercise and URTI can be modeled in the form of a "J" curve.[2,3] (See Figure 2.2). This model suggests that although the risk of URTI may decrease below that of a sedentary individual when one engages in moderate exercise training, risk may rise above average during periods of excessive amounts of high-intensity exercise. At present, there is more evidence, primarily epidemiological in nature, exploring the relationship between heavy exertion and infection. Much more research using larger subject pools and improved research designs is necessary before this model can be wholly accepted or rejected.

The model in Figure 2.2 also suggests that immunosurveillance mirrors that relationship between infection risk and exercise workload. In other words, it makes sense that if regular moderate exercise lowers infection risk, it should be accompanied by enhanced immunosurveillance. On the other hand, when an athlete engages in unusually heavy exercise workloads (e.g., overtraining or a competitive endurance race event), infection risk should be related to diminished immunosurveillance.[12]

Do the immune systems of endurance athletes and nonathletes function differently? Laurel Mackinnon has provided a review of this topic in Chapter 1. Although the URTI epidemiological data suggest that disparities should exist, attempts thus far to compare resting immune function in athletes and nonathletes have failed to provide compelling evidence that athletic endeavor is linked to clinically important changes in immunity.[13-17] The few studies available suggest that the innate immune system responds differentially to the chronic stress of intensive exercise, with natural killer cell activity tending to be enhanced while neutrophil function is suppressed (but only during unusually heavy periods of training).[2-4,13-15] The adaptive immune system (resting state) in general seems to be largely unaffected by athletic endeavor.

Even when significant changes in the concentration and functional activity of immune parameters have been observed in athletes, investigators have had little success in linking these to altered rates of infection and illness.[1-4,14,15,18] Of all immune cells, natural killer cells appear to be most affected by athletic endeavor — but in a positive way. In other words, the elevated natural killer-cell function often reported in athletes should enhance host protection against certain types of viruses and cancer cells. Neutrophils are an important component of the innate immune

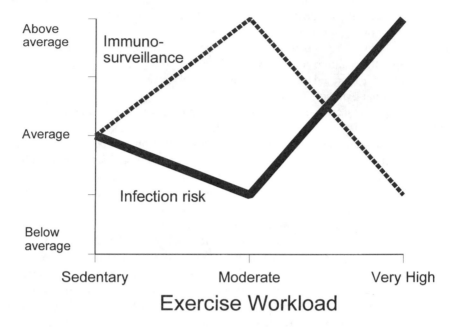

Figure 2.2 This model indicates that moderate exercise workloads are associated with improved immunosurveillance and decreased upper respiratory tract infection risk, while unusually high exercise workloads are associated with decreased immuno-surveillance and increased infection risk.

system, aiding in the phagocytosis of many bacterial and viral pathogens, and the release of immunomodulatory cytokines. Neutrophils are critical in the early control of invading infectious agents. In one report, elite swimmers undertaking intensive training had significantly lower neutrophil oxidative activity at rest than age- and sex-matched sedentary individuals, and function was further suppressed during the period of strenuous training prior to national-level competition.[15] Nonetheless, URTI rates did not differ between the swimmers and sedentary controls. Nieman et al.[14] reported that URTI rates were similar in female elite rowers and nonathletes during a 2-month period (winter/spring) despite higher natural killer function in the rowers (but normal granulocyte function). Salivary IgA concentration warrants further research as a marker of potential infection risk in athletes. Gleeson et al.[19] reported that salivary IgA levels measured in swimmers before training sessions showed significant correlations with infection rates, and the number of infections observed in the swimmers was predicted by the pre-season and the mean pre-training salivary IgA levels.

2.3 PROLONGED INTENSIVE EXERCISE AND IMMUNITY

Several authors have theorized that comparing resting immune function in athletes and nonathletes is not as important as measuring the magnitude of change in immunity that occurs after each bout of prolonged exercise.[4, 18, 20] During this "open window" of altered immunity (which may last between 3 and 72 hours, depending on the immune measure), viruses and bacteria may gain a foothold, increasing the risk of subclinical and clinical infection.

Although this is an attractive hypothesis, no serious attempt has been made by investigators to demonstrate that athletes showing the most extreme immunosuppression following heavy exertion are those that contract an infection during the following 1–2 weeks. This link must be established before the "open window" theory can be wholly accepted.

During the past decade, a plethora of research worldwide has greatly increased our understanding of the relationship between prolonged intensive exercise, the immune system, and host protection against viruses and bacteria.[1–4] Many components of the immune system exhibit change after heavy exertion, including the following:[4, 18]

- Neutrophilia (high blood neutrophil counts) and lymphopenia (low blood lymphocyte counts), induced by high plasma catecholamines, growth hormone, and cortisol

Exercise is associated with an extensive perturbation of white blood cell counts, with prolonged, high-intensity endurance exercise leading to the greatest degree of cell trafficking (increase in blood granulocyte and monocyte counts, and a decrease in blood lymphocytes).[21–24] Several mechanisms appear to be involved, including exercise-induced changes in stress hormone and cytokine concentrations, body temperature changes, increases in blood flow, lymphocyte apoptosis, and dehydration.[18, 21, 25–27] Following prolonged running at high intensity, the concentration of serum cortisol is significantly elevated above control levels for several hours, and has been related to many of the cell trafficking changes experienced during recovery.[4, 28] Demargination of neutrophils from the lung vasculature and the recruitment of neutrophils from the bone marrow contribute to the surge of neutrophils into the blood compartment following heavy exertion. Lymphocytes are recruited largely from the spleen into the blood compartment before exiting to sites yet undetermined.

- Increase in blood granulocyte and monocyte phagocytosis, but a decrease in nasal neutrophil phagocytosis

Following prolonged high-intensity running, substances released from injured muscle cells initiate an inflammatory response.[29–33] Monocytes and neutrophils invade the inflamed area, and phagocytose debris. The increase in blood granulocyte and monocyte phagocytosis might therefore represent a part of the inflammatory response to acute muscle injury. Phagocyte specimens collected from the peripheral blood, however, will possibly react differently from those taken from the respiratory tract. Using nasal lavage samples, Müns et al.[34] showed that the capacity of phagocytes to ingest *E. coli* was significantly suppressed in athletes for more than three days after running a 20-km road race compared with controls.

- Decrease in granulocyte oxidative burst activity

Although not an entirely consistent finding, granulocytes have a small but significant decrease in oxidative burst capacity following sustained heavy exertion.[35–37] The decrease in granulocyte oxidative burst may represent a reduced killing capacity by blood neutrophils (on a per cell basis) due to stress and overloading.[17]

- Decrease in nasal mucociliary clearance

In one report, nasal mucociliary transit time was significantly prolonged after heavy exertion, taking several days to return to normal.[38] These data, combined with the impairment in nasal neutrophil function and nasal/salivary IgA secretion rates, suggest that host protection in the upper airway passages is suppressed for a prolonged time after endurance running races.

- Decrease in natural killer-cell cytoxic activity (NKCA)

Following intensive and prolonged endurance exercise, NKCA is decreased 40%–60% for at least six hours.[4, 23, 39, 40] This decrease is greater and longer lasting than what has been reported for exercise of less than 1 h duration.[41] The decrease in NKCA appears to be related to the cortisol-induced redistribution of blood NK lymphocytes from the blood compartment to other tissues.[4] The activity of each NK cell appears to be normal, but the mass loss of NK cells from the blood compartment to sites yet undetermined reduces overall blood NK cell activity. The clinical significance of this finding is currently under investigation.

- Decrease in mitogen-induced lymphocyte proliferation (a measure of T cell function)

Compared with resting nonathletic controls, whole blood Con A-induced lymphocyte proliferation falls 30–40% (unadjusted for changes in T cell number) for more than 3 h following 2.5 h of intensive running.[22] Others have reported an even greater decrease after endurance-race events.[23, 42] The decrease in T cell function is more prolonged than has been described after exercise of less than 1 h duration.[4]

- Decrease in the delayed-type hypersensitivity response

In one report, the delayed-type hypersensitivity (DTH) reaction in the skin was suppressed two days after a competitive endurance race.[43] This indicates an impairment in a complex immunological process that involves several different cell types (including T cells) and chemical mediators.[43]

- Increase in plasma concentrations of pro- and anti-inflammatory cytokines (e.g., tumor necrosis factor alpha (TNF-α), interleukin-1 beta (IL-1-β), interleukin-6 (IL-6), interleukin-10 (IL-10), and interleukin-1 receptor antagonist (IL-1ra))

Cytokines are low-molecular-weight proteins and peptides that help control and mediate interactions among cells involved in immune responses. Exercise bouts that induce muscle cell injury cause a sequential release of the pro-inflammatory cytokines (TNF-α, IL-1-β, and IL-6, followed very closely by anti-inflammatory cytokines such as IL-10 and IL-1ra).[26, 32, 44-55] The changes are very similar to those that occur in response to physical trauma and inflammation.[31] Moderate exercise (e.g., brisk walking) does not induce a significant increase in blood cytokine levels.

- Decrease in ex vivo production of cytokines (interferon gamma (IFN-γ), TNF-α, IL-1, IL-2, IL-6, and IL-10) in response to mitogens and endotoxin

Several investigators have reported that the mitogen-induced release of various cytokines is suppressed after prolonged and strenuous exercise.[53, 55, 56] This finding is difficult to interpret because plasma levels of some of these cytokines (e.g., IL-6 and IL-10) are increased following heavy exertion, while separated blood immune cells have a reduced capacity for cytokine production. This may imply that immune cells from other sites (e.g., the muscle and other metabolically active areas) are producing the cytokines.

- Decrease in nasal and salivary IgA concentration

The secretory immune system of the mucosal tissues of the upper respiratory tract is considered the first barrier to colonization by pathogens, with IgA the major effector of host defense.[57,58] Secretory IgA inhibits attachment and replication of pathogens, preventing their entry into the body. Data from Müns et al.[59] have shown that IgA concentration in nasal secretions is decreased by nearly 70% for at least 18 hours after racing 31 kilometers. Following strenuous prolonged exercise, salivary IgA output falls, decreasing the level of IgA-mediated immune protection at the mucosal surface.[57, 60, 61]

- Blunted major histocompatibility complex (MHC) II expression and antigen presentation in macrophages

The major histocompatibility complex (MHC) antigens are essential for reactions of immune recognition. Class I MHC antigens play a role in self- and nonself recognition, while class II MHC antigens, found on antigen-presenting cells such as macrophages, assist in the process of cell-mediated immune responses. After phagocytosis and antigen processing, small antigenic peptides are bound to MHC II and presented to T lymphocytes, an important step in adaptive immunity. Exhaustive exercise (2–4 h per day for 7 days) significantly suppresses the expression of MHC II and antigen presentation in mice macrophages, an effect due in part to elevated cortisol levels.[62,63] These data imply that heavy exertion can blunt macrophage expression of MHC II, negatively affecting the process of antigen presentation to T lymphocytes, and thus their ability to respond to an antigenic challenge (e.g., DTH).

Taken together, these data suggest that the immune system is suppressed and stressed, albeit transiently, following prolonged endurance exercise.[4, 18, 64] These immune changes do not occur following moderate exercise. Thus, it makes sense (but still remains unproven) that URTI risk may be increased when the endurance athlete goes through repeated cycles of heavy exertion, has been exposed to novel pathogens, and experienced other stressors to the immune system including lack of sleep, severe mental stress, malnutrition, or weight loss.[2, 14]

To counter this increased risk of URTI, athletes should consider these guidelines.[2–4]

- Keep other life stresses to a minimum (mental stress in and of itself has been linked to increased URTI risk).
- Eat a well-balanced diet to keep vitamin and mineral pools in the body at optimal levels.
- Avoid overtraining and chronic fatigue.
- Obtain adequate sleep on a regular schedule (disruption linked to suppressed immunity).
- Avoid rapid weight loss (linked to adverse immune changes).
- Avoid putting the hands to one's eyes and nose (a major route of viral self-innoculation).
- Before important race events, avoid sick people and large crowds whenever possible.
- For athletes competing during the winter, an influenza vaccination is recommended.

2.4 NUTRITIONAL COUNTERMEASURES FOR EXERCISE-INDUCED INFLAMMATION AND IMMUNE ALTERATIONS

Although endurance athletes may be at increased risk for URTIs during heavy training cycles, they must exercise intensively to compete successfully. Athletes appear less interested in reducing training workloads, and more receptive to ingesting drugs or nutrient supplements that have the potential to counter exercise-induced inflammation and immune alterations.

There is some preliminary data that various immunomodulator drugs may afford athletes some protection against inflammation, negative immune changes, and infection during competitive cycles, but much more research is needed before any of these can be recommended.[65–67] Indomethacin, which inhibits prostaglandin production, has been administered to athletes prior to exercise, or used *in vitro* to determine whether the drop in NKCA can be countered. Although some success has been reported following 1 h of intensive cycling, indomethacin has been found to have no significant effect in countering the steep drop in NKCA following 2.5 h of running.[39] Other anti-inflammatory medications have not yet been adequately investigated.

Researchers have measured the influence of nutritional supplements, primarily zinc,[68] dietary fat,[69] vitamin C,[6–8, 70] glutamine,[71–78] and carbohydrate[11,35,40,49,79–85] on the immune and infection response to intense and prolonged exercise.[64,86,87] Chapters 3 through 7 of this book summarize current information on lipids, protein, glutamine, vitamins, and minerals. A brief overview will be provided in this chapter, with an emphasis on carbohydrate supplementation.

Several double-blind placebo studies of South African ultramarathon runners have demonstrated that 3 weeks of vitamin C supplementation (about 600 mg/day) is related to fewer reports of URTI symptoms.[6–8] This has not been replicated, however, by other research teams. Himmelstein et al.,[88] for example, reported no alteration in URTI incidence among 44 marathon runners and 48 sedentary subjects randomly assigned to a 2-month regimen of 1000 mg/day of vitamin C or placebo. A double-blind, placebo-controlled study was unable to establish that vitamin C supplementation (1,000 mg/day for 8 days) had any significant effect in altering the immune response to 2.5 h of intensive running.[70] More research is needed to sort out these contradictory findings. (See Chapter 6 for more detail).

Glutamine, a nonessential amino acid, has attracted much attention by investigators.[64,76,87] It is an important fuel, along with glucose, for lymphocytes and monocytes, and decreased amounts have a direct effect in lowering proliferation rates of lymphocytes. Reduced plasma glutamine levels have been observed in response to various stressors, including prolonged exercise.[71,76,79] Whether exercise-induced reductions in plasma glutamine levels are linked to impaired immunity and host protection against viruses in athletes is still unsettled, but the majority of studies have not favored such a relationship.[74,76,77,89] (See Chapter 5 for further information).

2.4.1 Influence of Carbohydrate on Immune Changes Following Heavy Exertion

Research during the 1980s and early 1990s established that a reduction in blood glucose levels was linked to hypothalamic–pituitary–adrenal activation, an increased release of adrenocorticotrophic hormone and cortisol, increased plasma growth hormone, decreased insulin, and a variable effect on blood epinephrine levels.[90,91] Given the link between stress hormones and immune responses to prolonged and intensive exercise,[4,82] a hypothesis has been proposed that carbohydrate, compared with placebo ingestion, should maintain plasma glucose concentrations, attenuate increases

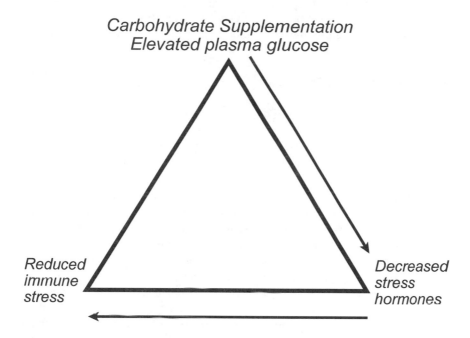

Figure 2.3   This model indicates that carbohydrate, compared with placebo supplementation during prolonged exercise, is associated with higher plasma glucose levels, an attenuated rise in plasma stress hormone concentrations, and reduced stress to the immune system.

in stress hormones, and thereby diminish changes in immunity (as summarized in Figure 2.3).

2.4.2.1   Research on Marathon Runners

This hypothesis was first tested in a group of 30 experienced marathon runners.[35,40,48,81] A double-blind, placebo-randomized study was designed to investigate the effect of carbohydrate fluid (6% carbohydrate beverage) ingestion on the immune response to 2.5 h of running. Marathoners in both groups averaged 11.9±0.2 km/h during the 2.5-h run at a heart rate of 151±2 beats/ min or 85.5±0.5% of the maximum heart rate, and an oxygen uptake of 40.9±0.8 ml·kg–¹· min–¹ or 76.7±0.4% of VO_{2max}. Drinking the carbohydrate beverage before, during (1 liter/h), and after 2.5 h of running attenuated the rise in both cortisol and the neutrophil/lymphocyte ratio.[35] The immediate post-run blood glucose level was significantly higher in the carbohydrate vs placebo group and was negatively correlated with cortisol ($r=-0.67$, $P<0.001$).[35] Trafficking of most leukocyte and lymphocyte subsets was lessened in accordance with the lower cortisol levels in the carbohydrate subjects.[35,40,81] Carbohydrate intake also blunted the rise in IL-6 and IL1-ra, cytokines involved in the inflammatory cascade response to heavy exertion.[48] Overall, these data supported the viewpoint that carbohydrate ingestion during prolonged and intensive exercise lessens hormonal and immune responses that have been related to physiological stress and inflammation. This was a striking finding, demonstrating that the stereo-typical immune changes that occur following heavy exertion lasting longer than 90 minutes could be altered by ingesting about 1 liter of carbohydrate beverage per h of exercise.

2.4.2.2 Research on Triathletes

In a subsequent study of 10 triathletes, carbohydrate ingestion was studied for its effect on the immune response to 2.5 h of running and cycling.[49,80,84] During four sessions (spread throughout a 4–6 week period), subjects ran on treadmills or cycled using their own bicycles on electromagnetically braked tripod trainers for 2.5 h at ~75% VO_{2max}. Subjects exercised under carbohydrate (6% carbohydrate beverage) or placebo conditions (double-blinded) (same as the prior experiment with the marathon runners). Sessions were assigned in a random, counterbalanced order. Carbohydrate or placebo beverages were ingested before, during (4 ml·kg^{-1} every 15 minutes of the 2.5-h exercise bout), and after exercise.

Carbohydrate, compared with placebo ingestion (but not activity mode), was associated with higher post-exercise plasma glucose levels and lower plasma con-centrations of cortisol and growth hormone.[49,80,84] For both modes, the placebo vs carbohydrate condition resulted in significantly higher blood concentrations of neu-trophils throughout recovery. Immediately post-exercise, monocytes and lympho-cytes (both NK and T cells) were higher in the placebo conditions, with lymphocytes falling markedly lower from 1.5 h to 3 h post-exercise.[84] As a result, the neutro-phil/lymphocyte ratio was elevated in the placebo conditions for both modes through-out recovery.[84] In parallel with the elevated NK cell counts immediately following exercise in the placebo vs carbohydrate condition, NKCA was also elevated, before falling below pre-exercise levels during recovery for both conditions.[49]

Plasma IL-6 levels following exercise were affected by both carbohydrate inges-tion and exercise mode, with levels after the carbohydrate cycling trial about one-fifth those measured after the placebo running trial.[49] Unlike IL-6, IL-1ra was not affected by exercise mode, but was decreased during several hours of recovery by about 60% after carbohydrate ingestion relative to placebo.[49] Figure 2.4 summarizes the IL-6 and IL-1ra data for the running trials by these triathletes. Bruunsgaard et al.[44] have shown that exercise involving eccentric muscle activity is associated with a much higher IL-6 response than concentric exercise. In another study in which muscle biopsies and blood samples were collected before and after a marathon race,[32] mRNA for IL-6 was detected in muscle but not in blood (where mRNA for IL-1ra was measured). These findings indicate that exercise-induced injury of muscle fibers in the skeletal muscles triggers local production of IL-6 (probably stimulated by TNF-α and IL-1β)that stimulates the production of IL-1ra from blood mononuclear cells. The data from the triathlete study are consistent with these findings, and further suggest that production of IL-1ra (and by association, IL-1β) after intensive exercise is affected by carbohydrate ingestion independent of exercise mode, probably through linkage to plasma cortisol levels. Cortisol and catecholamines have been related to the cytokine response to heavy exertion.[92]

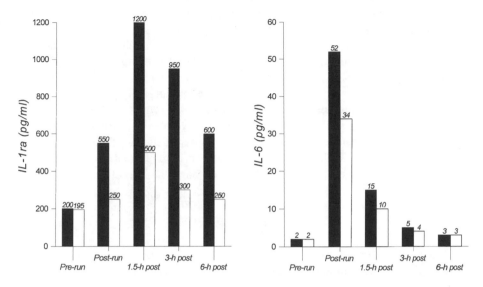

Figure 2.4   The pattern of change in plasma IL-1ra and IL-6 over time was significantly influenced by carbohydrate vs placebo ingestion in this study of 10 triathletes who ran for 2.5 h at high intensity.[49] (Black bars represent carbohydrates and white placebos.)

For 6 h following the running and cycling bouts, an increase in blood granulocyte and monocyte phagocytosis was measured, with levels somewhat lower following the carbohydrate trials (pre- to 3 h post-exercise increases were 40–48% for the carbohydrate trials vs 64–84% for the placebo trials).[84] Cortisol has been linked to enhanced phagocytosis, and thus it is likely that the lower phagocytic activity associated with carbohydrate ingestion in the triathletes was related to the lower cortisol levels induced by higher plasma glucose concentrations.[84] Carbohydrate ingestion also diminished the increase in granulocyte and monocyte oxidative burst activity following exercise.

2.4.2.3   Research on Rowers

In a third study, the influence of carbohydrate vs placebo beverage consumption on the immune and hormonal responses to normal rowing training sessions was measured in 15 elite female rowers residing at the U.S. Olympic Training Center.[83,93,94] In a randomized, counterbalanced design, the athletes received carbohydrate or placebo beverages (double-blinded) before, during, and after two 2-h bouts of rowing (1 day apart). Blood samples were collected before, and 5–10 min and 1.5 h after rowing. Metabolic measures indicated that training was performed at moderate intensities, with some high-intensity intervals interspersed throughout the sessions (mean workload, 57% of VO_{2max}).

Glucose and insulin were significantly lower after 2 h of rowing with ingestion of placebo compared with carbohydrate. The patterns of change in cortisol, growth hormone, epinephrine, and norepinephrine, however, did not differ between rowing trials. Blood neutrophil cell counts and the neutrophil/lymphocyte ratio, IL-1ra, and granulocyte phagocytosis were significantly higher following placebo vs carbohydrate rowing sessions, but the differences were not remarkable. The patterns of change in blood lymphocyte and lymphocyte subset counts, lymphocyte proliferative responses, IL-6, and salivary IgA did not differ between trials.[83,93,94] These data suggest that when exercise intensity is moderate, and changes in blood hormone and immune parameters are minimal, carbohydrate has a relatively minor influence. Together, these three studies indicate that carbohydrate ingestion plays a more important role in attenuating changes in immunity when the athlete experiences physiologic stress and depletion of carbohydrate stores in response to high-intensity ($\sim$75–80% VO_{2max}) exercise bouts lasting longer than 2 h.

2.5 CONCLUSIONS

Many components of the immune system exhibit adverse change after prolonged heavy exertion. These immune changes occur in several compartments of the immune system and body (e.g., the skin, upper respiratory tract mucosal tissue, lung, blood, and muscle). Although still open to interpretation, most exercise immunologists believe that during this "open window" of impaired immunity (which may last between 3 and 72 h, depending on the immune measure), viruses and bacteria may gain a foothold, increasing the risk of subclinical and clinical infection.

Can nutritional supplements serve as countermeasures to these immune changes following heavy exertion? Several nutritional supplements have been studied, primarily zinc, vitamin C, glutamine, and carbohydrate. Vitamin C and glutamine have received much attention, but the data thus far are inconclusive. The most impressive results have been reported with carbohydrate supplementation.

Carbohydrate beverage ingestion has been associated with higher plasma glucose levels, an attenuated cortisol and growth hormone response, fewer perturbations in blood immune cell counts, lower granulocyte and monocyte phagocytosis and oxidative burst activity, and a diminished pro- and anti-inflammatory cytokine response. Overall, these data indicate that the physiological stress to the immune system is reduced when endurance athletes use carbohydrate beverages before, during, and after prolonged and intense exertion. The clinical significance of these carbohydrate-induced effects on the endocrine and immune systems awaits further research.

REFERENCES

1. Hjertman, J.M.E, and Nieman, D.C., *Compendium of the Exercise Immunology Literature, 1997–1999*, Paderborn, Germany, International Society of Exercise and Immunology, 1999.
2. Nieman, D.C., Exercise immunology: practical applications, *Int. J. Sports Med.*, 18, S91,1997.

3. Nieman, D.C., Effects of athletic training on infection rates and immunity, in *Overtraining In Sport*, Kreider, R.B., Fry, A.C., and O'Toole, M., Eds., Human Kinetics, Champaign, IL,1998.
4. Nieman, D.C., Immune response to heavy exertion, *J. Appl. Physiol.*, 82, 1385, 1997.
5. Nieman, D.C., Johanssen, L.M., Lee, J.W., Cermak, J., and Arabatzis, K., Infectious episodes in runners before and after the Los Angeles Marathon, *J. Sports Med. Phys. Fitness*, 30, 316, 1990.
6. Peters-Futre, E.M., Vitamin C, neutrophil function, and URTI risk in distance runners: the missing link, *Exerc. Immunol. Rev.*, 3, 32, 1997.
7. Peters, E.M., Goetzsche, J.M., Grobbelaar, B., and Noakes, T.D., Vitamin C supplementation reduces the incidence of postrace symptoms of upper-respiratory-tract infection in ultramarathon runners, *Am. J. Clin. Nutr.*, 57, 170, 1993.
8. Peters, E.M., Goetzsche, J.M., Joseph, L.E., and Noakes, T.D., Vitamin C as effective as combinations of anti-oxidant nutrients in reducing symptoms of upper respiratory tract infection in ultramarathon runners, *S. Afr. J. Sports Med.*, 11(3), 23, 1996.
9. Nieman, D.C., Henson, D.A., Gusewitch, G., Warren, B.J., Dotson, R.C., Butterworth, D.E., and Nehlsen-Cannarella, S.L., Physical activity and immune function in elderly women, *Med. Sci. Sports Exerc.*, 25, 823, 1993.
10. Nieman, D.C., Nehlsen-Cannarella, S.L., Henson, D.A., Butterworth, D.E., Fagoaga, O.R., and Utter, A., Immune response to exercise training and/or energy restriction in obese women, *Med. Sci. Sports Exerc.*, 30, 679, 1998.
11. Nieman, D.C., Nehlsen-Cannarella, S.L., Markoff, P.A., Balk-Lamberton, A.J., Yang, H., Chritton, D.B.W., Lee, J.W., and Arabatzis, K., The effects of moderate exercise training on natural killer cells and acute URTIs, *Int. J. Sports Med.*, 11, 467, 1990.
12. Foster, C., Monitoring training in athletes with reference to overtraining syndrome, *Med. Sci. Sports Exerc.*, 30, 1164, 1998.
13. Nieman, D.C., Buckley, K.S., Henson, D.A, Warren, B.J., Suttles, J., Ahle, J.C., Simandle, S., Fagoaga, O.R., and Nehlsen-Cannarella, S.L., Immune function in marathon runners versus sedentary controls, *Med. Sci. Sports Exerc.*, 27, 986, 1995.
14. Nieman, D.C., Nehlsen-Cannarella, S.L., Fagoaga, O.R., Henson, D.A., Shannon, M., Hjertman, J.M.E., Bolton, M.R., Austin, M.D., Schilling, B.K., Schmitt, R., and Thorpe, R., Immune function in female elite rowers and nonathletes, *Br. J. Sports Med.* (in press).
15. Pyne, D.B., Baker, M.S., Fricker, P.A., McDonald, W.A., Telford, R.D., and Weidemann, M.J., Effects of an intensive 12-wk training program by elite swimmers on neutrophil oxidative activity, *Med. Sci. Sports Exerc.*, 27, 536, 1995.
16. Smith, J.A., Gray, A.B., Pyne, D.B., Baker, M.S., Telford, R.D., and Weidemann, M.J., Moderate exercise triggers both priming and activation of neutrophil subpopulations, *Am. J. Physiol.*, 270 (*Regulatory Integrative Comp. Physiol.*, 39), R838, 1996.
17. Smith, J.A. and Pyne, D.B., Exercise, training, and neutrophil function, *Exerc. Immunol. Rev.*, 3, 96, 1997.
18. Pedersen, B.K., Bruunsgaard, H., Klokker, M., Kappel, M., MacLean, D.A., Nielsen, H.B., Rohde, T., Ullum, H., and Zacho, M., Exercise-induced immunomodulation: possible roles of neuroendocrine and metabolic factors, *Int. J. Sports Med.*, 18, S2, 1996.
19. Gleeson, M., McDonald, W.A., Pyne, D.B., Cripps, A.W., Francis, J.L., Fricker, P.A., and Clancy, R.L., Salivary IgA levels and infection risk in elite swimmers, *Med. Sci. Sports Exerc.*, 31, 67, 1999.
20. Shephard, R.J. and Shek, P.N., Heavy exercise, nutrition and immune function: is there a connection?, *Int. J. Sports Med.*, 16, 491, 1995.

21. Haq, A., Al-Hussein, K., Lee, J., and al Sedairy, S., Changes in peripheral blood lymphocyte subsets associated with marathon running, *Med. Sci. Sports Exerc.*, 25, 186, 1993.

22. Nieman, D.C., Simandle, S., Henson, D.A., Warren, B.J., Suttles, J., Davis, J.M., Buckley, K.S., Ahle, J.C., Butterworth, D.E., Fagoaga, O.R., and Nehlsen-Cannarella, S.L., Lymphocyte proliferative response to 2.5 hours of running, *Int. J. Sports Med.*, 16, 404, 1995.

23. Shinkai, S., Kurokawa, Y., Hino, S., Hirose, M., Torii, J., Watanabe, S., Shiraishi, S., Oka, K., and Watanabe, T., Triathlon competition induced a transient immunosuppressive change in the peripheral blood of athletes, *J. Sports Med. Phys. Fitness*, 33, 70, 1993.

24. Suzuki, K., Naganuma, S., Totsuka, M., Suzuki, K.J., Mochizuki, M., Shiraishi, M., Nakiji, K., and Sugawara, K., Effects of exhaustive endurance exercise and its one-week daily repetition on neutrophil count and functional status in untrained men, *Int. J. Sports Med.*, 17, 205, 1996.

25. Brenner, I., Shek, P.N., Zamecnik, J., and Shephard, R.J., Stress hormones and the immunological responses to heat and exercise, *Int. J. Sports Med.*, 19, 130, 1998.

26. Gannon, G.A., Rhind, S.G., Suzui, M., Shek, P.N., and Shephard, R.J., Circulating levels of peripheral blood leucocytes and cytokines following competitive cycling, *Can. J. Appl. Physiol.*, 22, 133, 1997.

27. Kappel, M., Hansen, M.B., Diamant, M., Jørgensen, J.O.L., Gyhrs, A., and Pedersen, B.K., Effects of an acute bolus growth hormone infusion on the human immune system, *Horm. Metab. Res.*, 25, 579, 1993.

28. Cupps, T.R. and Fauci, A.S., Corticosteroid-mediated immunoregulation in man, *Immunol. Rev.*, 65, 133, 1982.

29. Belcastro, A.N., Arthur, G.D., Albisser, T.A., and Raj, A.J., Heart, liver, and skeletal muscle myeloperoxidase activity during exercise, *J. Appl. Physiol.*, 80, 1331, 1996

30. Bury, T.B. and Pirnay, F., Effect of prolonged exercise on neutrophil myeloperoxidase secretion, *Int. J. Sports Med.*, 16, 410, 1995.

31. Evans, W.J. and Cannon, J.G., The metabolic effects of exercise-induced muscle damage, *Exerc. Sport Sci. Rev.*, 19, 99, 1991.

32. Ostrowski, K., Rohde, T., Zacho, M., Asp, S., and Pedersen, B.K., Evidence that interleukin-6 is produced in human skeletal muscle during prolonged running, *J. Physiol. (Lond.)*, 508,(Pt 3), 949, 1998.

33. Raj, D.A., Booker, T.S., and Belcastro, A.N., Striated muscle calcium-stimulated cysteine protease (calpain-like) activity promotes myeloperoxidase activity with exercise, *Pflugers Arch.*, 435, 804, 1998.

34. Müns, G., Effect of long-distance running on polymorphonuclear neutrophil phagocytic function of the upper airways, *Int. J. Sports Med.*, 15, 96, 1993.

35. Nieman, D.C., Fagoaga, O.R., Butterworth, D.E., Warren, B.J., Utter, A., Davis, J.M., Henson, D.A., and Nehlsen-Cannarella, S.L., Carbohydrate supplementation affects blood granulocyte and monocyte trafficking but not function following 2.5 hours of running, *Am. J. Clin. Nutr.*, 66, 153, 1997.

36. Sato, H., Abe, T., Kikuchi, T., Sato, H., Abe, T., Kikuchi, T., Endo, T., Hasegawa, H., Suzuki, K., Nakaji, S., Sugawara, K., and Ohta, S., Changes in the production of reactive oxygen species from neutrophils following a 100-km marathon, *Nippon Eiseigaku Zasshi*, 51, 612, 1996.

37. Suzuki, K., Sato, H., Kikuchi, T., Abe, T., Nakaji, S., Sugawara, K., Totsuka, M., Sato, K., and Yamaya, K., Capacity of circulating neutrophils to produce reactive oxygen species after exhaustive exercise, *J. Appl. Physiol.*, 81, 1213, 1996.

38. Müns, G., Singer, P., Wolf, F., and Rubinstein, I., Impaired nasal mucociliary clearance in long-distance runners, *Int. J. Sports Med.,* 16, 209, 1995.
39. Nieman, D.C., Ahle, J.C., Henson, D.A., Warren, B.J., Suttles, J., Davis, J.M., Buckley, K.S., Simandle, S., Butterworth, D.E., Fagoaga, O.R., and Nehlsen-Cannarella, S.L., Indomethacin does not alter the natural killer cell response to 25 hours of running, *J. Appl. Physiol.,* 79, 748, 1995.
40. Nieman, D.C., Henson, D.A., Garner, E.B., Butterworth, D.E., Warren, B.J., Utter, A., Davis, J. M., Fagoaga, O.R., and Nehlsen-Cannarella, S.L., Carbohydrate affects natural killer cell redistribution but not activity after running, *Med. Sci. Sports Exerc.,* 29, 1318, 1997.
41. Woods, J.A., Davis, J.M., Smith, J.A., and Nieman, D.C., Exercise and cellular innate immune function, *Med. Sci. Sports Exerc.,*31, 57, 1999.
42. Eskola, J., Ruuskanen, O., Soppi, E., Viljanen, M.K., Jarvinen, M., Tolvonen, H., and Kouvalainen, K., Effect of sport stress on lymphocyte transformation and antibody formation, *Clin. Exp. Immunol.,* 32, 339, 1978.
43. Bruunsgaard, H., Hartkopp, A., Mohr, T., Konradsen, H., Heron, I., Mordhorst, C.H., and Pedersen, B.K., *In vivo* cell-mediated immunity and vaccination response following prolonged, intense exercise, *Med. Sci. Sports Exerc.,* 29, 1176, 1997.
44. Bruunsgaard, H., Galbo, H., Halkjaer-Kristensen, J., Johansen, T.L., MacLean, D.A., and Pedersen, B.K., Exercise-induced increase in serum interleukin-6 in humans is related to muscle damage, *J. Physiol.,* 499, (Pt 3), 833, 1997.
45. Bury, T.B., Louis, R., Radermecker, M.F., and Pirnay, F., Blood mononuclear cell mobilization and cytokines secretion during prolonged exercises, *Int. J. Sports Med.,* 17, 156, 1996.
46. Drenth, J.P., Van Uum, S.H.M., Van Deuren, M., Pesman, G.J., Van der Ven-Jongekrijg, J., and Van der Meer, J.W., Endurance run increases circulating IL-6 and IL-1ra but down regulates *ex vivo* TNFα and IL-1β production, *J. Appl. Physiol.,* 79, 1497, 1995.
47. Dufaux, B. and Order, U., Plasma elastase-α1-antitrypsin, neopterin, tumor necrosis factor, and soluble interleukin-2 receptor after prolonged exercise, *Int. J. Sports Med.,* 10, 434, 1989.
48. Nehlsen-Cannarella, S.L., Fagoaga, O.R., Nieman, D.C., Henson, D.A., Butterworth, D.E., Bailey, E., Warren, B.J., and Davis, J.M., Carbohydrate and the cytokine response to 2.5 hours of running, *J. Appl. Physiol.,* 82, 1662, 1997.
49. Nieman, D.C., Nehlsen-Cannarella, S.L., Fagoaga, O.R., Henson, D.A., Utter, A., Davis, J.M., Williams, F., and Butterworth, D.E., Influence of mode and carbohydrate on the cytokine response to heavy exertion, *Med. Sci. Sports Exerc.,* 30, 671, 1998.
50. Northoff, H., Weinstock, C., and Berg, A., The cytokine response to strenuous exercise, *Int. J. Sports Med.,* 15, S167, 1994.
51. Ostrowski, K., Rohde, T., Asp, S., Schjerling, P., and Pedersen, B.K., Pro- and anti-inflammatory cytokine balance in strenuous exercise in humans, *J. Physiol. (Lond.),* 1999, 515(Pt 1), 287.
52. Rohde, T., MacLean, D.A., Richter, E.A., Kiens, B., and Pedersen, B.K., Prolonged submaximal eccentric exercise is associated with increased levels of plasma IL-6, *Am. J. Physiol.,* 273(1 Pt 1), E85, 1997.
53. Smits, H.H., Grunberg, K., Derijk, R.H., Sterk, P.J., and Hiemstra, P.S., Cytokine release and its modulation by dexamethasone in whole blood following exercise, *Clin. Exp. Immunol.,* 111, 463, 1998.

54. Sprenger, H., Jacobs, C., Nain, M., Gressner, A. M., Prinz, H., Wesemann, W., and Gemsa, D., Enhanced release of cytokines, interleukin-2 receptors, and neopterin after long-distance running, *Clin. Immunol. Immunopath.*, 63, 188, 1992.

55. Weinstock, D., Konig, D., Harnischmacher, R., Keul, J., Berg, A., and Northoff, H., Effect of exhaustive exercise stress on the cytokine response, *Med. Sci. Sports Exerc.*, 29, 345, 1997.

57. Mackinnon, L.T, and Hooper, S.L., Mucosal (secretory) immune system responses to exercise of varying intensity and during overtraining, *Int. J. Sports Med.*, 15, S179, 1994.

58. Nieman, D.C. and Nehlsen-Cannarella, S.L., The effects of acute and chronic exercise on immunoglobulins, *Sports Med.*, 11, 183, 1991.

59. Müns, G., Liesen, H., Riedel, H., and Bergmann, K-Ch., Einfluß von langstreckenlauf auf den IgA-gehalt in nasensekret und speichel, *Deut. Zeit. Sportmed.*, 40, 63, 1989.

60. Ljungberg, G., Ericson, T., Ekblom, B., and Birkhed, D., Saliva and marathon running, *Scand. J. Med. Sci. Sports*, 7, 214, 1997.

61. Steerenberg, P.A., van Asperen, I.A., van Nieuw Amerongen, A., Biewenga, A., Mol, D., and Medema, G.J., Salivary levels of immunoglobulin A in triathletes, *Eur. J. Oral Sci.*, 105, 305, 1997.

62. Woods, J.A., Ceddia, M.A., Kozak, C., and Wolters, B.W., Effects of exercise on the macrophage MHC II response to inflammation, *Int. J. Sports Med.*, 18, 483, 1997.

63. Ceddia, M.A. and Woods, J.A., Exhaustive exercise decreases macrophage antigen presentation, *J. Appl. Physiol.*, (in press).

64. Pedersen, B.K., Ostrowski, K., Rohde, T., and Bruunsgaard, H, Nutrition, exercise and the immune system, *Proc. Nutr. Soc.*, 57, 43, 1998.

65. Atalay, M., Marnila, P., Lilius, E.M., Hanninen, O., and Sen, C.K., Glutathione-dependent modulation of exhausting exercise-induced changes in neutrophil function of rats, *Eur. J. Appl. Physiol.*, 74, 342, 1996.

66. Ghighineishvili, G.R., Nicolaeva, V.V., Belousov, A.J., Sirtori, P.G., Balsamo, V., Miani, A, Franceschini, R., Ripani, M., Crosina, M., and Cosenza, G., Correction by physiotherapy of immune disorders in high-grade athletes, *Clin. Ter.*, 140, 545, 1992

67. Lindberg, K. and Berglund, B., Effect of treatment with nasal IgA on the incidence of infectious disease in world-class canoeists, *Int. J. Sports Med.*, 17, 235, 1996.

68. Singh, A., Failla, M.L., and Deuster, P. A., Exercise-induced changes in immune function: effects of zinc supplementation, *J. Appl. Physiol.*, 76, 2298, 1994.

69. Venkatraman, J.T. and Pendergast, D., Effect of the level of dietary fat intake and endurance exercise on plasma cytokines in runners, *Med. Sci. Sports Exerc.*, 30, 1198, 1998.

70. Nieman, D.C., Henson, D.A., Butterworth, D.E., Warren, B.J., Davis, J.M., Fagoaga, O.R., and Nehlsen-Cannarella, S.L., Vitamin C supplementation does not alter the immune response to 2.5 hours of running, *Int. J. Sports Nutr.*, 7, 174, 1997.

71. Castell, L.M. and Newsholme, E.A., The effects of oral glutamine supplementation on athletes after prolonged, exhaustive exercise, *Nutrition*, 13, 738, 1997.

72. Castell, L.M., Poortmans, J.R., Leclercq, R., Brasseur, M., Duchateau, J., and Newsholme, E.A., Some aspects of the acute phase response after a marathon race, and the effects of glutamine supplementation, *Eur. J. Appl. Physiol.*, 75, 47, 1997.

73. Castell, L.M., Poortmans, J.R., and Newsholme, E.A., Does glutamine have a role in reducing infections in athletes?, *Eur. J. Appl. Physiol.*, 73, 488, 1996.

74. Mackinnon, L.T. and Hooper, S.L., Plasma glutamine and upper respiratory tract infection during intensified training in swimmers, *Med. Sci. Sports Exerc.*, 28, 285, 1996.

75. Rohde, T., Ullum, H., Rasmussen, J.P., Halkjaer Kristensen, J., Newsholme, E., and Pedersen, B.K., Effects of glutamine on the immune system: influence of muscular exercise and HIV infection, *J. Appl. Physiol.*, 79, 146, 1995.

76. Rohde, T., Krzywkowski, K., and Pedersen, B.K., Glutamine, exercise, and the immune system—is there a link?, *Exerc. Immunol. Rev.*, 4, 49, 1998.

77. Rohde, T., MacLean, D.A., and Pedersen, B.K., Effect of glutamine supplementation on changes in the immune system induced by repeated exercise, *Med. Sci. Sports Exerc.*, 30, 856, 1998.

78. Rowbottom, D.G., Keast, D., Goodman, C., and Morton, A.R., The haematological, biochemical and immunological profile of athletes suffering from the overtraining syndrome, *Eur. J. Appl. Physiol.*, 70, 502, 1995.

79. Gleeson, M., Blannin, A.K., Walsh, N.P., Bishop, N.C., and Clark, A.M., Effect of low- and high-carbohydrate diets on the plasma glutamine and circulating leukocyte responses to exercise, *Int. J. Sport Nutr.*, 8, 49, 1998.

80. Henson, D.A., Nieman, D.C., Blodgett, A.D., Butterworth, D.E., Utter, A., Davis, M.J., Sonnenfeld, G., Morton, D.S., Fagoaga, O. R., and Nehlsen-Cannarella, S.L., Influence of exercise mode and carbohydrate on the immune response to prolonged exercise, *Int. J. Sports Nutr.*, 9, 221, 1999.

81. Henson, D.A., Nieman, D.C., Parker, J.C.D., Rainwater, M.K., Butterworth, D.E., Warren, B.J., Utter, A., Davis, J.M., Fagogaga, O.R., and Nehlsen-Cannarella, S.L., Carbohydrate supplementation and the lymphocyte proliferative response to long endurance running, *Int. J. Sports Med.*, 19, 1, 1998.

82. Nieman, D.C., Influence of carbohydrate on the immune response to intensive, prolonged exercise, *Exerc. Immunol. Rev.*, 4, 64, 1998.

83. Nieman, D.C., Nehlsen-Cannarella, S.L., Fagoaga, O.R., Henson, D.A., Shannon, M., Davis, J.M., Austin, M.D., Hjertman, J.M.E., Bolton, M.R., Schilling, B.K., Hisey, C., and Holbeck, J., Immune response to two hours of rowing in female elite rowers, *Int. J. Sports Med.*, 20, 476, 1999.

84. Nieman, D.C., Nehlsen-Cannarella, S.L., Henson, D.A., Utter, A., Davis, J.M., Williams, F., and Butterworth, D.E., Influence of carbohydrate ingestion and mode on the granulocyte and monocyte response to heavy exertion in triathletes, *J. Appl. Physiol.*, 84,1252, 1998.

85. Mitchell, J.B., Pizza, F.X., Paquet, A., Davis, B.J., Forrest, M. B., and Braun, W.A., Influence of carbohydrate status on immune responses before and after endurance exercise, *J. Appl. Physiol.*, 84, 1917, 1998.

86. Newsholme, E.A., Biochemical mechanisms to explain immunosuppression in well-trained and overtrained athletes, *Int. J. Sports Med.*, 15, S142, 1994.

87. Shephard, R.J. and Shek, P.N., Immunological hazards from nutritional imbalance in athletes, *Exerc. Immunol. Rev.*, 4, 22, 1998.

88. Himmelstein, S.A., Roberbs, R.A., Koehler, K.M., Lewis, S.L., and Qualls, C.R., Vitamin C supplementation and upper respiratory tract infections in marathon runners, *J.E.P.$_{online}$*, 1(2), 1, 1998.

89. Shewchuk, L.D., Baracos, V.E., and Field, C.J., Dietary L-glutamine does not improve lymphocyte metabolism or function in exercise-trained rats, *Med. Sci. Sports Exerc.*, 29, 474, 1997.

90. Mitchell, J.B., Costill, D.L., Houmard, J.A., Flynn, M.G., Fink, W.J., and Beltz, J.D., Influence of carbohydrate ingestion on counterregulatory hormones during prolonged exercise, *Int. J. Sports Med.*, 11, 33, 1990.

91. Murray, R., Paul, G.L., Seifent, J.G., and Eddy, D.E.. Responses to varying rates of carbohydrate ingestion during exercise, *Med. Sci. Sports Exerc.,* 23, 713, 1991.
92. Papanicolaou, D.A., Petrides, J.S., Tsigos, C., Bina, S., Kalogeras, K.T., Wilder, R., Gold, P.W., Deuster, P.A., and Chrousos, G.P., Exercise stimulates interleukin-6 secretion: inhibition by glucocorticoids and correlation with catecholamines, *Am. J. Physiol.,* 271, (3 Pt 1), E601, 1996.
93. Henson, D.A, Nieman, D.C., Nehlsen-Cannarella, S.L., Fagoaga, O.R., Shannon, M., Bolton, M.R., Davis, J.M., Gaffney, C.T., Kelln, W.J., Austin, M.D., Hjertman, J.M.E., and Schilling, B.K., Influence of carbohydrate ingestion on cytokine and phagocytic responses to two hours of rowing, *Med. Sci. Sports Exerc.,* (in press).
94. Nehlsen-Cannarella, S.L., Nieman, D.C., Fagoaga, O.R., Kelln, W.J., Henson, D.A., Shannon, M., and Davis, J.M., Salivary immunoglobulins in elite female rowers, *Eur. J. Appl. Physiol.,* 81, 222, 2000.

CHAPTER 3

LIPIDS, EXERCISE, AND IMMUNOLOGY

Jaya T. Venkatraman, Peter J. Horvath, and David R. Pendergast

CONTENTS

1-8493-0741-4/00/$0.00+$.50
© 2000 by CRC Press LLC

3.1 INTRODUCTION

The role of lipids on the immune responses to exercise has been under appreciated. This is due in large part to the relatively recent advances in immunology. In addition, the "fat phobia" in athletes, particularly female athletes, and their advisers has resulted in an over-emphasis on the role of carbohydrates during exercise and the failure to recognize the importance of glycogen sparing by fat oxidation. Nutritionists also believe that a high-fat diet may compromise the immune system. Recent studies have established the potential role of fat oxidation in glycogen sparing,[1] and in fact, have shown that increasing the fat intake in athletes can increase exercise endurance and in some athletes maximal aerobic power.[2-4] The purpose of this chapter is to show how a low-fat diet might compromise the immune system, and how a higher-fat diet might improve it. Consideration will be given to exercise and dietary lipids, and how these two factors, together, affect the immune system.

3.2 EXERCISE

3.2.1 Acute and Chronic Exercise

The term "exercise" should be defined prior to an examination of its interaction with the immune system and dietary lipids. Acute exercise has to be considered a "stressor" as it results in increased metabolism, excess heat production, and widespread physiological adjustments.[1] If exercise is carried out routinely (chronic exercise), the body can adapt (training effect) and eliminate or raise the threshold of the stress imposed by exercise. Chronic exercise that is too stressful, however, leads to decompensation of the body (overtraining). This overtraining is often associated with consumption of fewer total calories than expended and intake of fewer fats than needed.[5] Nutritional imbalances result in depletion of intramuscular energy stores of glycogen and fats. The combination of these overstresses and reduced energy stores may result in increased stress to the immune system during exercise training and performance.

3.2.2 Intensity and Duration of Exercise

The intensity and duration (time) of exercise determine the level of stress imposed on the body and thus, the physiological and immunological responses. The exercise intensity determines the neuromuscular, metabolic, cardiopulmonary, and neurohumoral responses. These responses are graded to the exercise intensity when slow-twitch muscle fibers are recruited and oxidative mechanisms are used. The recruitment of fast-twitch muscle fibers during higher-intensity exercise, above maximal aerobic power, requires anaerobic–glycolytic energy; the stresses imposed are significantly elevated. At a given exercise intensity, the capability to sustain the effort as a function of time (duration) adds additional physiological and metabolic stress. There is an inverse relationship between exercise duration and exercise intensity. The intensity of exercise determines the rate of energetic pathways used to resynthesize adenosine triphosphate (ATP) and thus, determine substrate use. The duration of the exercise determines the total amount of substrates used and, specifically, the amount of intramuscular glycogen and fats. The availability of these substrates influences the athlete's endurance, and their absence could increase the stress of exercise on the immune system.

3.2.3 Substrate Use

Carbohydrates and fats are the two main fuels that are metabolized in the muscle to provide energy (ATP) for muscular contraction. Their relative contribution to energy expenditure during exercise depends on various factors such as intensity and duration of the exercise, the diet before exercise, and training. During prolonged exercise (more than 2 h), fat is the major form of fuel, which may exceed 90% in extreme circumstances.[6] People who are able to oxidize more fat at a certain work-load or speed (endurance-trained athletes) can exercise longer at a higher intensity. This indicates that the capacity to oxidize fat is a major determinant of endurance exercise performance. Before fatty acids can be oxidized, they must be mobilized and transported to the site of oxidation. At rest, about 70% of all free fatty acids are reesterified.[7] During exercise, reesterification is suppressed, and the rate of lipolysis is accelerated, resulting in large amounts of free fatty acids (FFA) in blood.[8] Triglycerides (TG) bound to lipoproteins are also a potential source of fatty acids.[9] The enzyme lipoprotein lipase in the vascular wall will hydrolyze some of the TG in the circulating lipoproteins passing through the capillary bed. This results in FFA release that the muscles can use for oxidation.

Fats taken up and oxidized from the blood can provide 20%–30% of the total fat oxidized from low to maximal aerobic exercise, respectively.[10] The remaining 70%–80% of fat oxidized comes from the intramuscular fat stores. These intramuscular fat stores are in droplets that are in contact with the mitochondria. These fat stores become depleted during endurance exercise.[11]

3.2.4 Fat Utilization

When exercise is initiated, the rate of fat oxidation from the intramuscular fat droplet increases, and the rates of lipolysis and FFA release from adipose tissue are increased. During the first 15 min of exercise, FFA concentrations decrease. Thereafter, the rate of appearance of FFA will depend on the utilization by muscles. Fat oxidation increases during endurance exercise. Fat oxidation will be high during low-intensity (60–70%VO_2 max) exercise. Carbohydrates are the main fuel source during high-intensity exercise, although fat oxidation still plays an important role, particularly in slow-twitch fibers.

3.2.5 Effects of Training

Endurance training affects substrate utilization and exercise capacity. Several studies have established a marked adaptive increase in oxidative potential in response to an increased physical activity.[12] Enhanced exercise capacity after endurance training is probably due to the shift of metabolism to a greater use of fat and a concomitant sparing of glycogen reserves.[13] Endurance training may result in adaptations such as increases in the number of mitochondria, amount of oxidative enzymes, mitochondrial contents, TG oxidation, FFA uptake, alterations in the mobilization of FFAs from adipose tissue, and increased stores of intramuscular fats.[6]

Early studies have demonstrated that endurance exercise performance is dependent on intramuscular glycogen stores.[1] It has also been shown that decreasing the amount of carbohydrates in the diet to 20% of total calories and increasing the amount of fat to 60%–75% (balance protein) in the diet, either during or recovery from exhaustive exercise, resulted in a significant reduction in exercise performance.[14] Furthermore, supplementing athletes with carbohydrates during endurance exercise increased the athletes' endurance.[15] These studies were supported by techniques to measure intramuscular levels of glycogen. Similar studies to determine the role of intramuscular fat were not undertaken. The combination of the results of these studies led to the overall conclusion that fats were not essential in endurance performance and that the important fuel was carbohydrates. This conclusion was confounded by observations that the amount of energy needed to run a marathon could not be provided by glycogen alone, and that athletes had considerably greater ability to oxidize fats, and thus, spare glycogen.

In more-recent studies, endurance capacity has been shown to be lower on a diet low in fat (15% of total calories) than on a 32% fat diet, and higher on diets with 42%–54% fat.[2, 16, 17] These findings have been reported for exercise intensities of 60%–80% of maximal aerobic power. In these studies, some of the participants had a 5%–10% increase in maximal aerobic power, as well as the increased endurance capacity.[2] A limitation of these studies was that the total caloric intake of the athletes on low-fat diets was about 800 Kcal less than expended and what could be sustained on the higher-fat diets. Correcting the caloric deficit with carbohydrates increased endurance performance about 10%. However, increasing the deficit with fats increased endurance performance by 20%.[16] The explanation for the improved endurance performance is in the amount of fats and carbohydrates stored in the muscle. An examination of the intramuscular fat deposits in runners showed a 60% increase of intramyocellular fat on a 42%-fat diet than on a 15%-fat diet, without a significant reduction in intramuscular glycogen.[11] The increased fat oxidation during endurance exercise spared glycogen, and allowed the runner to run longer prior to glycogen/fat depletion.

The conclusion from these studies is that reducing fat intake to very low levels compromises exercise performance, and increasing the amount of fat in the diet and the total caloric intake may improve performance. These observations are particularly true in female athletes, who as a consequence of low caloric intake, low fat intake, and high energy expenditure, have markedly altered neuro-hormonal function, including amenorrhea.

The stresses imposed by exercise may have an impact on immune function as circulating levels of epinephrine, norepinephrine, and cortisol in the blood are increased. In addition, the ability to repair muscle damage, due directly to mechanical factors or secondarily to oxidative stress, may be influenced by the individual's immune status. The immune function may be related to the balance between amount and type of fat in the diet and the utilization of fat as a fuel during exercise.

3.3 DIETARY LIPIDS

3.3.1 Lipid Components

The lipids that exist in the diet in the greatest amount (more than 95%) are triglycerols (TG: both fats and oils). The human diet can also contain substantial amounts of phospholipids and sterols. Also consumed by humans are numerous other lipid-soluble materials, such as fat-soluble vitamins and many antioxidants, that may have physiological actions during exercise and affect the immune responses. Many features of fatty acids should be considered when studying the effect of lipids on exercise and the immune system. These include chain length, degree of unsaturation, and the double bonds' location and geometry. Chain length and degree of unsaturation may affect absorption and metabolism (oxidation and storage). The geometry, in terms of cis or trans configuration and the distance between the double bonds, could have profound effects on metabolism. The most prominent sterol in most human diets is cholesterol, but many individuals, especially those who avoid dietary fat, consume much higher amounts of phytosterols.

Many dietary components either coexist with the more common lipids or require them for optimal absorption. Some of these may be vitamins (vitamin E or vitamin-like coenzyme Q10), pharmacological agents (antioxidants like the carotenoids), or have hormone-like actions (phytochemicals like the isoflavones). Additionally, some unusual lipid-soluble components have been studied as ergogenic aids (e.g., octacosanol).

3.3.2 Dietary Lipid Intake

3.3.2.1. Total Caloric Intake

The total caloric expenditure in male and female athletes is two- to threefold that of sedentary individuals due to the increased level of daily exercise in training and performing. In spite of the high caloric expenditure, studies in both male and female runners have reported that their caloric intakes are only 65%–75% of their estimated caloric expenditure.[18–21] Estimated caloric expenditure may be in error, but there is little doubt that athletes in general are in caloric deficits and that many are on diets low in fat.[5, 20, 22–24] Increasing the fat intake of runners from 15%–42% increased their total caloric intake by 17%–26% and brought them near energy balance.[16] Although many athletes purposely reduce their fat and total caloric intake to maintain a low body weight, increasing fat from 15%–42%, or total calories by 25%, did not result in an increase in body weight or percentage of body fat.[16]

Protein intake in the diets of most athletes is sufficient to meet the demands (0.8 g/kg/day).[16] The percentage of fat in the diet can be increased to 42%, with a protein intake of 20% and a carbohydrate intake of 38%. This is sufficient to maintain intramuscular glycogen stores on a calorically balanced diet. Conversely, on a high-carbohydrate diet (65%), with 20% protein, the fat intake (15%) on a low-calorie diet is not likely to maintain intramuscular fats stores. This may be the reason that endurance performance was reduced in male and female runners (20%) who were on a low-fat diet.[2]

Vitamins A, E, and C may serve as protective antioxidants in athletes, who, due to their higher energy expenditures, may have greater oxidative stress. Athletes are generally above the Recommended Dietary Allowances (RDA) levels in these vitamins, however, only on a high-fat diet[16] do they achieve levels that have been suggested to improve antioxidant capacity.[25] Iron intake is lower on a low-fat diet, particularly in women, than on a high-fat diet. In addition, calcium is below RDA[20, 26] on low-fat diets, but exceeded it on high-fat diets. Zinc status is increased on high-fat diets, however runners are still below the RDA levels.[20, 26]

In conclusion, the self-selected low-fat diets that many athletes eat may not be the most beneficial in terms of energy, essential fatty acids, vitamin E, calcium, and zinc intake. This is particularly true as low-fat diets are almost always associated with a caloric intake that is less than caloric expenditure, leading to reduced intramuscular stores of substrate and reduced exercise performance. The reduction of these essential fats, vitamins, and minerals and intramuscular energy stores may also compromise immune function.

3.3.2.2 Total Dietary Fat Intake

The intake of dietary fat has been decreasing over the past decade. Paradoxically, obesity has been on the rise in the past decades. The typical intake of fat in the U.S. is about 37% of total calorie intake. The dietary fat intake by athletes training for various sports events is summarized in Table 3.1. Most high-caliber athletes attempt to restrict fat intake, but most studies show that their fat intakes, as a percentage of energy intake, are not much different from the general populace. With female athletes, vegetarians are more likely to consume less dietary TG.[45] Low dietary fat intake has been related to hormone irregularities, such as reduced prolactin levels and amenorrhea.[45] Many other factors related to low fat intake, such as high dietary fiber intake, low energy intake, and low protein intake, may contribute to hormone irregularities. Elevated levels of dietary fiber can increase fecal estrogen output.[46] Low energy intake may result in an adaptive loss of luteal function.[47, 48]

Saturated fatty acids (SFAs) account for nearly 15% of the total caloric intake in the U.S. diet.[49] Major sources of these SFAs include animal fat, chocolate, coconut oil, and palm oil. The two former sources are much higher in stearic acid (18:0) while the two later sources are high in shorter SFA. Stearic acid is metabolized more like oleic acid (18:1) than the shorter SFA. Some of the shorter SFA are in the range of medium chain fatty acids, which can be used to synthesize medium chain triglycerides (MCT). These have been studied as a unique energy source and have been found to be digested, absorbed, and transported differently from the long-chain fatty acids. In addition, they are metabolized in the mitochondria like long-chain fatty acids, but they do not require transport into the mitochondria by carnitine transferase.

Monounsaturated fatty acids (MUFAs) compose approximately 15% of the total caloric intake in the U.S. diet. They are derived from animal fat and vegetable oils (olive and canola). Most commonly occurring MUFAs exist in the cis form, but

Table 3.1 Fat Intake in Athletes Training for Various Sports Events

Population	Subjects	%Energy from Fat	Reference
Division 1 athletes	Figure Skaters	34	Grandjean, 1989[27]
	Wrestlers	34	
	Basketball Players	41	
Division 1 athletes	Average, many sports	36	Short & Short 1983 [28]
	Football players	40	Short & Short 1983 [28]
	Football players	39	Hickson et al, 1987b[29]
Female College Athletes	Many sports	42	Welch et al, 1987[30]
E. German elite athletes		39	Strauzenberg et al, 1987[31]
Australian Olympians	Male	43	
	Female	45	Steel, 1970[32]
Adolescent, professional school	Female dancers	35	Benson et al, 1985[20]
Adolescent, Canadian Olympic	Female field hockey	39	Ready, 1987[33]
High School	Football players	39	Hickson et al, 1987b[34]
Nordic Ski Team, U.S.	Male	38	Ellsworth et al, 1985[35]
	Female	37	
Dutch Olympic rowers		43	De Wijn et al, 1985[36]
Ultra distance runner, 500 km		26	Manore et al, 1989[37]
Wheelchair marathoners		26	Lally et al, 1991[38]
Olympic marathoners	Female	32	Deuster et al, 1986[39]
Nat. Soccer team	Puerto Rico	32	Rico et al, 1992[40]
Triathletes, Iron Man championship		30	Worme et al, 1990[45]
Triathletes, Australian		27	Burke & Read, 1987[43]
Bodybuilding championship,	USA	14	Bazarre et al, 1990[44]

Note: Typically, vegetarians consume less dietary TG than those eating meat.

microbial, animal, and industrially produced fats can contain high levels of trans fatty acids.

Many varied types of fatty acids make up the broad category of polyunsaturated fatty acids (PUFA). In the U.S., they account for about 7% of the total caloric intake. Two major classes of PUFAs exist: omega (ω)-6 and ω–3. ω-6 and ω–3 compose the fatty acids (ω–6 series: linoleic, arachidonic; ω–3 series: eicosapentanoic, EPA; and docosahexanoic acid, DHA). These are important as precursors of the second messenger eicosanoids. The major ω–6 fatty acid, linoleic acid, is found in high levels in vegetable oils. Increased consumption of linoleic acid has been promoted as a way to lower total plasma cholesterol. However, when linoleic acid is consumed in amounts greater than 10% of total calories, high-density lipoprotein cholesterol (HDL-C) could decrease while low-density lipoprotein (LDL) oxidation increases.[50, 51] High levels of linoleic acid could also suppress the immune system.[52] Eicosapentanoic acid (EPA) is the most prominent ω–3 fatty acid in cold-water fish (and fish oil); high levels of linolenic acid occur in some vegetable oils (evening primrose oil and flaxseed oil).

Cholesterol intake is less for women than men in the U.S. (300 vs. 400 mg/day).[53] Elite Nordic skiers have been reported to consume up to 1.2 g/day for males and 700 mg/day for females,[35] while professional soccer players consumed approximately 700 mg/day. Certain athletes (collegiate football players) may consume enormous levels of cholesterol, over 3400 mg/day, due to consumption of eggs.[28]

3.3.3 Fat Supplementation and Exercise

Dietary fats are slow in reaching the circulation because of delayed gastric emptying and digestion.[54] Long-chain fatty acids enter the blood 3–4 h after ingestion. MCT supplements may be effective during extreme endurance exercise when the reliance on blood substrate is maximal. Reduced fat and total caloric intake compromise maximal aerobic power and exercise endurance.[16, 17, 55] This observation can be corrected, in part, by increasing total caloric intake. However, the dietary fat intake had to be increased to 42% of total calories to maximize endurance performance in runners.[16, 17]

3.4 IMMUNE FUNCTION RELATED TO EXERCISE

The immunologic response to exercise comprises numerous alterations within the immune system, but how these processes are regulated is still largely unknown. Exercise-related immunological changes include signs of inflammation, such as release of inflammatory mediators, activation of various white blood cells and complement, and induction of acute-phase proteins (see Figure 3.1). Nevertheless, signs of immunosuppression, such as decreased T- and B-cell function or impaired cytotoxic or phagocytic activity, can also be observed. Without sufficient recovery, both single bouts of exhausting physical activity and chronic exercise (overtraining) may impair immune responses and increase an athlete's vulnerability to acute and chronic inflammation and reduced post-exercise tissue repair.[56, 57]

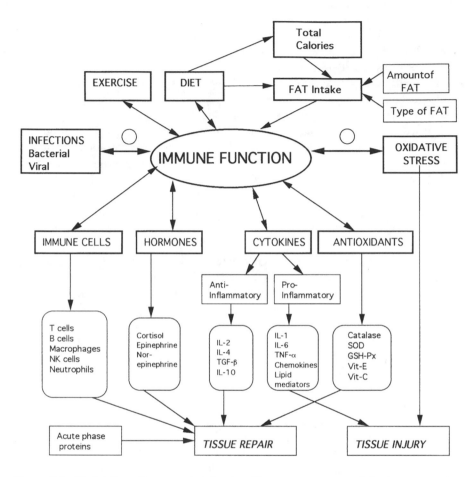

Figure 3.1   Modulation of immune function by different components of the immune system
and possible mechanisms through which dietary lipids and exercise may modulate
immune function. NK-natural killer cells; IL-interleukins; TGF-β-Transforming
Growth Factor-β; TNF-α-tumor necrosis factor-α; SOD-superoxide dismutase;
GSH-Px-Glutathione peroxidase; Vit-C-vitamin C; Vit-E- vitamin E.

The epidemiological data suggest that endurance athletes are at increased risk
for upper-respiratory-tract infections (URTI) during periods of heavy training and
the 1–2-week period following a marathon or similar events. After acute bouts of
prolonged heavy exercise, several components of the immune system are suppressed
for several hours.[58, 59] After prolonged intense exercise, the number of lymphocytes
in the blood is reduced, and the function of natural killer cells is suppressed;
furthermore, secretory immunity is impaired. During this time of immunodepression,
often referred to as "the open window," the host may be more susceptible to microorganisms bypassing the first line of defense. Clinical observations regarding an
increased risk of infections in top athletes are compatible with this model.[60]

The immune responses to the stresses of exercise involve coordination of many cell types, soluble factors, and messenger molecules in the blood and throughout the body. The modulation of immune function by different components of the immune system and the possible mechanisms through which dietary lipids and exercise may modulate immune function are summarized in Figure 3.1. Exercise causes marked changes in the number, proliferation, and distribution of circulating leukocytes. The level of dietary-fat intake, oxidative stress, certain hormones, cytokines, and types of immune cells may enhance proinflammatory effects of strenuous exercise. As both the type and amount of dietary fat can modulate immune function through modulating lymphoid cell subsets, secretion of pro-and anti-inflammatory cytokines etc., and through selecting the right amount and type of fat in the diet, it may be possible to overcome some of the negative effects of strenuous exercise on the immune system. The distribution of leukocytes has been attributed to hormonal regulation that occurs during, immediately following, and for long periods after exercise. The immune depression of the body in general, and, following severe exercise, the mucosal system, may be mediated by the effects of elevated body temperature, cytokines, and several stress-related hormones. Soluble factors such as cytokines are important in initiating and regulating the immune responses. Exercise-induced immunomodulation may occur due to altered composition of immunocompetent cells and activation of the immune system. Although exercise-induced effects on the immune system may be transient, the temporary changes could increase the vulnerability to infections, and if exercise is chronic and/or severe, may place these athletes at high risk.

Several researchers have implied that regular and moderate excrcise, where physiological adaptations accompany the training, may improve the ability of the immune system to protect the host from infection.[61–63] It is important that, to obtain maximal benefits from exercise, factors such as the total caloric intake, level of fat in the diet, and training level need to be balanced to obtain the optimal effect on the immune system, though a sound balance in the cytokines and hormones is essential. Runners with a more serious commitment to exercise experienced fewer infectious episodes than recreational runners who were less serious.[64] Whereas adaptations to exercise may protect the immune system, severe and prolonged exercise may compromise it physiologically, leading to exaggerated neurohormonal responses. In addition, there may be depletion of the energy stores, particularly fats, which are needed for exercise metabolism and maintenance of the immune system. These factors, considered together, could explain the compromised immune systems of athletes who are overstressed.

3.4.1 Lymphoid Cell Subsets

Mobilization of different leukocyte subsets during exercise has been reported.[65] Alterations of the different lymphocyte functions can be at least partly explained based on the changes observed in the subpopulations of peripheral blood mononuclear (PBMN) cells. Two possible mechanisms have been suggested for this pattern of responses. One possibility is that lymphocytes with a differing quantitative expression of surface marker antigen might be mobilized into the circulation from other body compartments following exercise. The other possibility is that the expression of these surface marker antigens might be up- or down-regulated by some unknown factors that are induced by exercise. In exercise of short duration, the former mechanism may be more likely. The effects of exercise of different intensity and duration in subjects with different fitness levels have been studied by several investigators; some of their results are summarized in Table 3.2. These studies generally report transient leukocytosis, lymphocytosis, and increased natural killer (NK) cell number and activity. However, different sports, performed at maximum intensity, induce different immune system changes.

The effect of intensive physical exercise on interleukin-1 (IL-1), tumor necrosis factor α (TNF- α), and certain lymphocyte subsets are proinflammatory (Figure 3.1) and are affected by exercise.[69] Interleukin-2 (IL-2) decreases immediately after exercise but increases after 24 h, compared with the pre-exercise values taken at steady state. TNF- α has been shown to increase 2 h after exercise, then return to habitual values after 24 h. Increases in NK cells are observed post exercise. The ratio of T-helper/T-suppressor (CD4$^+$/CD8$^+$) ratio is reduced to varying degrees based on the intensity of physical activity. This decrease is observed immediately after exercise, followed by increased ratios 2 h later, due to oppositely directed quantitative changes of the CD4$^+$ and CD8$^+$ cell populations. After 24 h, the ratios return to habitual levels.

Both high- and moderate-intensity exercise are associated with shifts in circulating proportions of NK cells, which influence interpretation of natural killer cytolytic activity (NKCA) data, based on assays using separated mononuclear cells.[74] Long-term running may induce some change in lymphocyte subpopulations.[75] Chronic submaximal exercise induces increased mobilization of neutrophils and decreased mobilization of lymphocytes, and decreases the absolute and relative number of neutrophils at rest.[44] Dietary lipid intervention may modulate lymphoid cell subsets, and thereby may alter proliferative response, cytokine production, etc., in pathological conditions such as autoimmune diseases, anorexia, etc. Hence, it is logical to presume that some of the negative or inflammatory effects of strenuous exercise can be corrected or minimized by selecting the appropriate fat level and the type of fat in the diet

3.4.2 Proliferative Response to Mitogens

While the number of lymphocytes in the blood may be elevated by physical exercise, their functions may be impaired. *In vitro* impairment of responses to mitogens has been associated with a variety of immune deficiencies *in vivo*, such as changes in CD4/CD8 ratios, decreases in the production of IL-2, increases in prostaglandin E$_2$ (PGE$_2$) levels, increases in macrophage function, etc. (Figure 3.1). The reduction in the CD4/CD8 ratio below 1.5 may decrease DNA synthetic responses. This reduced response may be sufficient to allow microorganisms and viruses time to evade early immunological recognition and establish ongoing infection in runners. Mitogen stimulation of T cells *in vitro*, using suboptimal doses, is believed to mimic events that occur after the antigen stimulation of T cells *in vivo*. Generally, moderate-intensity exercise will decrease the proliferative response by 35%–50%.[80]

Table 3.2. Effects of Exercise of Varying Intensities and Training on Lymphoid Cell Subsets in Human Subjects

Study	Subjects	Findings	Investigator
Prolonged exercise	16 male swimmers 17 non-swimmers	↑ in leukocytes, lymphocytes & NK cells	Boas et al. (1996)[66]
Elite swimmers	Elite swimmers	*After run:* ↑ in CD3, CD4, CD5, CD8, CD19, CD57, CD18, CD16/CD22, ↓ in prolif. resp. *24h after run:* Normal levels subsets, No change in plasma cytokines	Espersen et al. (1996)[67]
4 wks. aerobic training	Men-40–50yrs, mod. trained	*At rest:* ↓ in CD3, CD4 *4 wks. training:* ↓ in CD4, naive cells.	Weiss et al. (1995)[68]
5km run	Well-conditioned runners	*Imm. after:* ↓ in IL-2, CD4/CD8 ratio, inc. in TNF, HLA-DR+ cells, NK *24h after:*↑ in IL-2, normal TNF	Espersen et al. (1990)[69]
Endurance run	5 endurance runners (at 95%VO2)	*Imm. after:* ↓ in prolif resp., No changes in T & B cell functions, Inc. in NK, CD8+	Hinton et al. (1997)[70]
Aerobic Exercise (3– 45-min. cycling/10 wk)	Sedentary men-18–40yrs.	↑ in resting CD2, CD4, CD45RA+CD4+, CD8 & CD20	La Perriere et al. (1994)[71]
30-min. mod. exer.	Runners-25	*Imm. after:* T lymphocytosis, ↓ in CD4+/CD8+ratio, prolif. resp to PHA	Smith et al. (1993)[72]
Graded maximal exercise with hypoxia	Sedentary subjects did exercise	↑ in: CD3, CD4+, CD45RO-, CD45RO+, CD8+CD45RO-, CD8+CD45RO+, CD3-CD16/CD56+, CD3+CD16/CD56+, CD19, Adrenaline, noradrenaline, cortisol.	Gabriel (1993)[76]
Intensity (80%VO2 vs.. 50% VO2)	Young men-well cond-itioned,45min	*80% VO2: Imm. after:* ↑NK, NKCA *1–2h after:* ↓ in NK	Nieman et al. (1993)[74]
Long-term run (8-km 5xwk-40 wk)	Healthy men & women-20yrs	↑ in (suppressor/inducer), suppressor T cells, ↓ in Leu 3a+ Leu8- (cytotoxic T cells)	Kawada et a.l (1992)[75]
Intensive endurance	17 cyclists-20yrs	NK cells & naive CD8 cells get transported to injured muscles	Gabriel (1991)[76]
Intensity & duration	Men-defined fitness	↓ in resp. to Con-A,↑ in intensity → ↓ resp to Con-A	MacNeil (1991)[77]
Acute, chronic max. exer-6m	6-controls, 6-cyclists	Max. exercise: ↑ subsets, NK, CD8+	Ferry et a.l (1990)[78]
Intensity, duration & fitness	Healthy men	*Imm. after exercise:* ↓ in CD3+, CD4, Higher the fitness → Higher ↑ in NK	Hoffman-Goetz et a.l (1990)[79]

The decreased response to phytohemagglutinin-A (PHA) during exercise has been linked to a decreased proportion of T cells[81] or to an increased proportion of NK cells. When the proliferative response was adjusted on a per cell basis, no difference was observed in NK cell cytotoxicity or concanavalin-A (Con-A)-induced T cell proliferation.[82] Significant correlations between total mitogen response and the composition of the cultured lymphocytes has been reported.[70] A consistent depression in mitogenesis present 2 h after an exercise bout in all fitness groups has been reported.[77] The magnitude of the reduction in T-cell mitogenesis was not affected by an increase in exercise duration. A trend toward greater reduction in proliferative response was present in the highly fit group when exercise intensity was increased. The reduction in lymphocyte proliferation to concanavalin A after exercise was a short-term phenomenon with recovery to resting (pre-exercise) values 24 h after cessation of the exercise bout.

These data suggest that single sessions of submaximal exercise transiently reduce lymphocyte function in men and that this effect occurs irrespective of the subject's fitness level. The large increases in NK cells, relative to T-cells, following intensive exercise, were the most likely cause of the reduced mitogenic response of total lymphocyte cultures. Healthy human subjects 40 to 60 years old performing anaerobic training experienced, on average, a significant decrease of circulating $CD4^+$ T-lymphocytes, while other parameters, including CD8 and CD4, remained unchanged.[68] Post-exercise suppression of mitogenic responses to PHA is due to the release of serum factor(s) capable of inducing prostaglandin synthesis by circulating monocytes. Whereas exercise-induced suppression of pokeweed mitogen (PWM) responses depends primarily on the reversal of $CD4^+/CD8^+$ ratios,[72] both the quantity and type of fat are known to influence the proliferative response of immune cells to mitogens.

3.4.3 Cytokines

Various humoral messengers, including cytokines, hormones, and neurotransmitters, regulate cellular and humoral immunity (see Figure 3.1). Cytokines are important in initiating and regulating the immune response, influencing almost all immune functions. Cytokines, which various immunocompetent cells produce in response to appropriate stimuli, mediate many immune functions and orchestrate the immune system. They act as molecular signals between immunocompetent cells. The excessive or insufficient production of cytokines may contribute to infectious, immunological, and inflammatory diseases. Cytokines participate in several cellular, immunological, and inflammatory responses. A balance between pro- and anti-inflammatory cytokines is essential for the maintenance of a sound immune system.

Exercise can alter the release of numerous cytokines and modulate their receptor systems. Such changes may trigger inflammatory and acute-phase responses (see Figure 3.1). After high-intensity exercise, the immune system becomes involved in tissue repair processes. Increases in IL-1, IL-6 and TNF-α have been found in supernatants from LPS-stimulated PBMN cells isolated from untrained persons 2 h after bicycle exercise. Plasma IL-6 and TNF- α increase following long-distance running. Inflammation in athletes may be caused by mechanical stress, local ischemia, and/or free-radical generation in the active skeletal muscle. There is evidence suggesting that systemic elevation of cytokines occurs in serum after strenuous exercise. Suppression of IL-2 and increases in IL-1 and TNF- α production are reported after exercise.[76,83,84] Physical exercise, including eccentric muscle contractions, induces increases in the production of monokines. Elevations in plasma

IL-1 and TNF- α are thought to cause muscle proteolysis; IL-1 activity increased following eccentric exercise in untrained subjects.[85]

The underlying mechanisms of enhanced cytokine production during and after physical exercise remain unknown at present. The enhanced metabolism occurring during exercise may produce unknown intermediate products that are responsible for initiating leukocyte activation and cytokine release. Dietary lipids have an effect on cytokine balance, which is very critical for sound functioning of the immune system. Fish oil is known to lower the production of IL-1, IL-6 and TNF- α by macrophages. The effects of dietary lipids in modulating the levels of IL-2 and TGF-β under pathological conditions is known.

3.4.4 Neuroendocrine System

The immune system is closely linked to the neuroendocrine system. The magnitude and period of the leucocytosis, as mentioned earlier, depends on the intensity and duration of the workload. Neuroendocrine factors released in situations of stress, such as intense exercise, are suggested to be partly responsible for the exercise-induced changes in the immune system. Most immunosuppressive responses induced by intense exercise correlate with increases in circulating cortisol.[86, 87] It has been established that the leucocytosis induced by exercise is mediated by catecholamines and glucocorticoids,[88] and the specific immune response of lymphocytes is also mediated by adrenaline, glucocorticoids, β-endorphin, and other stress hormones.[89]

Exercise is known to activate the pituitary-adrenocortical axis to increase cortisol levels. At the present time, there are no reports on the effects of dietary fat on exercise-induced alterations and neuroendocrine hormone levels. Muscular exercise increases the concentrations of a number of stress hormones in the blood, including adrenaline, noradrenaline, growth hormone, beta-endorphins, and cortisol, whereas the concentration of insulin decreases slightly.[90] Stress hormones may play a role in mediating the exercise-related immunological changes. Adrenaline and noradrenaline may be responsible for the immediate effects of exercise on lymphocyte subpopulations and cytotoxic activities. Cortisol may be responsible for maintaining lymphopenia and neutrocytosis after exercise of long duration.[91]

A significant increase in the blood cortisol level usually requires a duration of exercise of more than 20 minutes above 60% of the VO_{2max}. It is primarily the consequence of a higher secretion rate.[92] Sustained cortisol secretion, up to a 200% increase, has been observed after a marathon run.[87] Plasma cortisol level is decreased with age in sedentary subjects, but is elevated in trained subjects across all age groups.[93] The magnitude of this increase in cortisol was substantially lower in trained subjects exercising at the same absolute workload as their untrained counterparts.[93]

3.4.5 Serum Soluble Immunoactive Markers

The activation of serum soluble immunoactive markers, such as soluble IL-2 receptors (sIL-2R), soluble intercellular adhesion molecule-1 (sICAM-1), soluble TNF-receptor (sTNF-R), and neopterin may be influenced by exercise.[94] Compared with baseline levels, all the parameters were significantly increased as a result of mountain climbing.[94] Within 36 h after the mountain climbing, sIL-2R, sCD8 and sICAM-1 decreased. In contrast, sTNF-R and neopterin levels remained higher than baseline throughout the study, only partially decreasing 24 and 36 h from start. These data showed immune-system activation induced by physical exercise. The increase of sTNF-R and neopterin, reflecting activation of macrophages, was sustained. The data suggest that immune activation phenomena may be involved in the pathogenesis of impaired immune function after exercise.

3.5 DIETARY FAT, EXERCISE, AND IMMUNE FUNCTION

3.5.1 Dietary Fat and Immune Function

It is generally accepted that increased fat in the diet is associated with immunocompetence. Exercise training may improve immune function; however, acute exercise or overtraining may compromise the immune system. Although high fat may improve performance, it could compromise immune function.[95-97] The mechanisms by which lipids may modulate immune function may involve several factors and mediators (see Figure 3.2).[97, 98] Both the quantity and type of dietary lipids are known to have modulator effects on the cellular immune system at the biochemical and molecular level, including the production and expression of cytokines.[99, 100] Dietary ω-6 lipids generally increase the levels of pro-inflammatory cytokines and inflammatory PGs, while ω-3 lipids may decrease the levels of these cytokines and inflammatory PGs[101-103] (See Figure 3.2).

Scientists now recognize that many metabolic processes respond directly or indirectly to pro-inflammatory cytokines. This cytokine-mediated "reprogramming" of metabolism is a homeorhetic mechanism that ensures an adequate supply of nutrients for proliferation of lymphocyte and macrophage populations, antibody production, and hepatic synthesis of acute-phase proteins. Pro-inflammatory cytokines have been linked to altered nutrient uptake and utilization. Anabolic processes are interrupted, and companion catabolic activities are amplified. Changing dietary fat consumption may alter the immune system and hormone levels, as lipids are components of biomembranes, serve as precursors for certain steroid hormones and prostaglandins, have a role in regulating eicosanoid synthesis, and interact directly with cellular activation processes.

Several mechanisms have been suggested to explain the action of dietary lipids, which are known to influence the fatty-acid composition of biological membranes. They are incorporated into the membrane lipid components, which mostly are phospholipids. The mechanisms by which lipids might modulate immune function could involve several factors and mediators.[95] Dietary ω-6 lipids (linoleic acid and linolenic acid present in vegetable oils such as corn oil and soybean oil) generally increase the levels of pro-inflammatory cytokines and inflammatory PGs, while long-chain ω-3 lipids (eicosapentanoic acid, docosahexanoic acid present in oil from marine sources such as fish oil) may decrease the levels of these cytokines and inflammatory prostaglandins.[95 98, 102] Thus, both the quality and quantity of dietary fat may modulate exercise-induced alterations on the immune system.[99, 102]

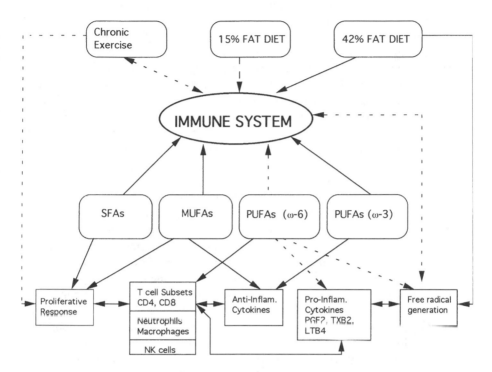

Figure 3.2 Possible mechanisms through which exercise and different types of dietary lipids may be modulating various components of the immune system. (→ positive effect and ⇢ negative effect); SFAs–saturated fats; MUFAs– Monounsaturated fats; PUFAs–Polyunsaturated fats; NK cells–natural killer cells.

The other known effects of ω–6 and ω–3 fatty acids are associated with the alteration in eicosanoid synthesis of PGs, thromboxanes (TXs), and leukotrienes (LTs). Under normal conditions, these eicosanoids are produced by the oxidation of arachidonic acid (AA, 20:4 ω–6). Desaturation of PUFAs is an important reaction to synthesize the very-long-chain fatty acids that are necessary for membrane functions and formation of eicosanoids. In general, the eicosanoids produced from AA are in the 2- and 4- series, such as PGE_2, PGI_2, TXA_2, and LTB_4. PGE_2 has a number of pro-inflammatory effects. In addition, PGs and other eicosanoids play a role in regulating the differentiation and functions of T-cells, B-cells, NK cells, and macrophages. In particular, TXA_2 can cause platelet aggregation that leads to thrombosis, PGI_2 can prevent platelet aggregation, and LTB_4 can attract neutrophils and eosinophils to inflammatory sites. PUFAs with 20 carbons are preferentially incorporated into tissue phospholipids with a relatively high specificity for AA.[104, 105]

3.5.2 Lipids And Cytokines

It is clear that cytokines affect whole-body nutrition and metabolism, and are responsible for many of the clinically observed nutritional effects of injury, infection, cancer, fever, hypermetabolism, anorexia, protein catabolism, cachexia, and altered fat, glucose, and trace mineral metabolism.[106] These metabolic and nutritional effects of cytokines are influenced by the nutritional status of the host, which is generally altered during the course of the critical illness. In the future, the use of specialized diets and the use of selective cytokine blockers are likely to be important components of the overall care of the catabolic patients. It is generally the PUFAs of the ω–6 series that increase the levels of proinflammatory cytokines and prostaglandins. Perhaps the types of fats in the diets are beneficial in preventing the exercise-induced rise in pro-inflammatory cytokines. As lipids are powerful mediators of the immune system, and they exert their effects on cytokines, hormones etc., the immunosuppressive effects of strenuous exercise can be modulated by carefully selecting both quality and quantity of dietary fats.

Some data suggest that essential fatty acids help regulate inflammatory processes, modulating both cytokine release and the acute-phase response. Positive effects of changing dietary essential fatty acids have been demonstrated in chronic inflammatory diseases.[107] In contrast, little is known about the contribution of the different fatty acids to the exercise-induced immunologic reaction. Essential fatty acids may determine alterations within the immune system following exercise.

Cytokines can decrease lipoprotein lipase and increase lipolysis in cultured fat cells. *In vivo,* many cytokines increase serum TG by increasing very-low-density lipoprotein production.[108] IFNs increase TG predominantly by decreasing lipoprotein lipase activity and TG clearance. These changes in lipid metabolism do not cause cachexia. Rather, they represent part of the host defense, as lipoproteins scavenge infectious particles such as endotoxin. IL-6 induces many of the endocrinologic and metabolic changes found in catabolic states and thus may mediate some of the metabolic effects previously ascribed to other cytokines.[109] Host-tumor interactions lead to a nonspecific inflammatory response mediated in part by the chronic production and release of proinflammatory cytokines, including IL-1, TNF-α, IL-6, and IFN-γ, which antagonize the anabolic signals associated with enteral and parenteral nutrition support.[110] Cytokine-mediated alterations can explain the inability of adequate dietary nitrogen and calories to result in lean tissue repletion. As the production of several cytokines is under negative control by PGE_2, synthesis of PGE_2 is decreased after consumption of ω–3 PUFA. A rise in PGE_2 may decrease IL-2 production and inhibit the response of T-cells to IL-2 and enhance IgG production by B cells or plasma cells.[111] Several investigators have studied the effect of the increased intake of these fatty acids on cytokine production.

Human studies reported to date have consistently demonstrated a decrease in the production of proinflammatory cytokines when moderate to high levels of marine-derived ω–3 PUFAs are taken orally.[99, 112] Production of IL-1β was assessed. *In vitro* production of IL-1 β and TNF-α in stimulated peripheral blood mononuclear cells (PBMCs) was reported to decrease after six weeks of ω–3 PUFA fish oil supplementation to male volunteers.[99] *In vitro* addition of EPA to human PBMCs is also reported to inhibit the production of IL-2 and the expression of the IL-2 receptor.[111, 113]

The influence of PGE_2 on the immune system has been explored to a limited extent. PGs of the E series are generally synthesized by macrophages and they suppress the lymphocyte response to T cell mitogens.[114] PGs released by monocytes after intense exercise inhibits NK cell function[115] and induced immune suppression.[116] Exercise causes some injuries in muscle and joints that may increase PGE_2 level.[117] Both the quantity and type of dietary fat are known to influence the level of PGE_2. It is known that high-fat diets tend to increase the level of plasma PGE_2. It is evident from studies from animal models that diets high in w-6 PUFAs generally increase plasma PGE_2 levels and PGE_2 production by lipopolysaccharide-stimulated macrophages.[118] This indicates that dietary fat may help reduce the stress caused by exercise and, therefore, has less or no adverse effects on well trained athletes who engage in exercise. Biomembranes serve barrier functions and as a store for precursors of rapidly generated, structurally diverse intracellular and extracellular lipid-derived mediators. Cytokines exert a dramatic multilevel impact in regulating enzymes in generating lipid-derived mediators central to their action.

3.6 INCREASING DIETARY FAT AND IMMUNE STATUS

3.6.1 Lymphoid Cell Subsets, Proliferative Response and *in Vitro* Production of Cytokines By PBMN Cells

The mechanism of action of dietary fat in modulating exercise-induced alterations on the immune system is not well understood. Increased endurance capacity in response to increasing dietary fat has been observed in both animal[119] and human studies.[120] The effects of three levels of dietary fat (low, medium, and high; 4 weeks on each diet) on the immune status of runners has been reported.[17] The dietary fat in these studies was distributed between saturated (40%), monounsaturated (37%), and polyunsaturated (23%) fats. The effects of these diets on peripheral blood mononuclear (PBMN) cell number, lymphoid cell subsets, proliferative response to lectins, and *in vitro* production of pro- and anti-inflammatory cytokines by PBMN cells (prior to and after a short bout of exhaustive exercise) was determined. An overall summary of the effects of increasing the levels of dietary fat on PBMN cell lymphoid cell subsets, proliferative response, and *in vitro* production of cytokines is presented in Table 3.3. In addition, the level of cytokines, hormones, and lipid peroxides was also determined in the plasma at rest and immediately after an all-out endurance run.

The percentage of NK^+ cells was increased by exercise from 3.9 ± 0.8 to 7.9 ± 1.2 for women and 4.1 ± 0.6 to 9.4 ± 1.3 for men with an increase in dietary fat (Figure 3.3). Exercise increased leukocyte cell counts, lymphocyte surface markers, CD8 (suppressor) for T cells, the number of NK cells, and decreased the level of IL-1 and $TNF\alpha$, especially in men. Increased dietary fat levels significantly increased anti-inflammatory cytokine IL-2 after exercise. Proliferative response to PWM by PBMN cells also decreased with the increase of dietary fat and exercise.

It may be possible to reduce the chronic stress on the immune system associated with overtraining through appropriately selecting the amount of dietary fat and matching total caloric intake to caloric expenditure. As both the quantity and quality of lipids are known to have immunomodulatory roles, it may be possible to overcome

Table 3.3 Effect of Dietary Lipids and a Short Intense Bout of Maximal Exercise on Peripheral Blood Mononuclear (PBMN) Cells[1] in Runners

	Max. Exercise	Gender	Diet Fat
Cell number[2]	↑	NE	NE
Lymphoid cell subsets:			
CD4+ (helper T cells)	NE	NE	NE
CD8+ (suppressor T cells)		higher (men)	↑(LF>MF)
CD14+ (monocytes)	NE	NE	NE
CD16 (NK cells)	↑	yes	yes
Proliferative response:[4]			
Con-A	NE	NE	NE
PHA	↑	lower (men)	↑
PWM	↓	lower (men)	↓
***In vitro* production of cytokines:[5]**			
IL-2 (PHA)	↑	men (higher)	↑
IL-1β (PWM)	NE	NE	↓
IL-6 (PWM)	↓	NE	↑
TNF-α (PWM)	↓	NE	↑

[1]PBMN cells were isolated by histopaque gradient centrifugation;[2]Viability of cells was tested by trypan blue exclusion;[3] Enumerated by flowcytometry;[4] Cells were cultured in the presence of optimal concentrations of lectins for 96 h and proliferative response was determined using MTT assay; Con-A–concanavalin A; PHA–phytohemagglutinin; PWM–pokeweed mitogen,[5]Cells were cultured in the presence of lectins and cytokines determined in cell free supernatants by ELISA; NE–no effect. Summarized from Venkatraman et al. (1997)[17]

the inflammatory effects of exercise by providing dietary lipids, which have a tendency to lower the inflammatory effect through modulating pro- and anti-inflammatory cytokines and free-radical generation. The observed decreases in the level of proinflammatory cytokines on a high-fat diet may be explained in part by the low levels of PUFA in the diets of the runners who participated in this study. In women runners, both medium- and high-fat diets significantly increased the number of NK cells and IL-2 levels over the levels of a low-fat diet. In the case of male runners, the high-fat diet lowered the proliferative response to PBMN cells to pokeweed mitogen (PWM) and increased IL-2 production over a low-fat diet. Saturated and monounsaturated fat levels were higher than polyunsaturated fats in all diets in these studies.[17] Recently, monounsaturated fatty acids have been reported to be less inflammatory than ω–6 fatty acids and oils such as olive oil, which are rich in monounsaturated fatty acids, e.g. oleic acid (18:1).

3.6.2 Plasma Cytokines and Hormones

Plasma IL-2 levels have been shown to be higher in male than female runners and to decrease in men with increased dietary fat. The level of plasma IFN-γ was independent of gender, exercise, and level of dietary fat. The plasma IL-6 level was lower after an exhaustive endurance run and decreased with an increase in the percent of dietary fat intake (Table 3.4). Increasing the level of dietary fat had no adverse effects on the level of plasma proinflammatory cytokines in runners.[121] Though endurance-run time increased with medium-fat and high-fat diets as compared with a low-fat diet, plasma IL-6 levels decreased after the exhaustive endurance run. A high-fat diet decreased plasma IL-6 levels in women after the endurance run. Both the exercise and high-fat diet increased the level of IL-2 and lowered the level of IL-6, suggesting that it is possible to modulate the level of specific proinflammatory cytokines through increased dietary fat intake, thus offsetting the proinflammatory effects of exercise.

Table 3.4 Effect of Dietary Lipids and Endurance on Plasma Cytokines and Hormones in Runners

	Endurance	Gender	Diet fat
Cytokines[1]			
IL-2		higher (men)	Men - Dec; Women - NE
IFN-γ	NE	NE	NE
IL-1β	NE	NE	NE
IL-6	$\downarrow$	NE	$\downarrow$
TNF-α	NE	NE	NE
Hormones[1]			
Cortisol	$\uparrow$	NE	Women–$\uparrow$; Men-NE
PGE2	$\uparrow$	NE	$\downarrow$
Lipid peroxides[2]	$\uparrow$	NE	$\downarrow$

[1]Plasma cytokines and hormones were quantitated by ELISA; [2]Lipid peroxides were determined using PerOxiquant kit. NE–no effect. Summarized from Venkatraman and Pendergast (1998),[122] and Feng, Pendergast, and Venkatraman (1997).[121]

The cortisol level was shown to be higher in women on a high-fat diet than on a low-fat diet (15% fat), but not in men. In male runners, the plasma cortisol level decreased on a medium-fat diet compared with a low-fat diet at rest and after exercise.[122, 123] In male runners, the PGE_2 level was higher when the runners were on a low-fat diet than when they were on the higher-fat diet. The data showed that the combined effects of high-fat diets and exercise are different from the effect of dietary fat and exercise analyzed separately. No significant increase in plasma cortisol, PGE_2 and IFN-γ levels were observed on a high-fat diet of well trained athletes after an exhaustive endurance run. It appears that increasing dietary fat can increase endurance-run time without adverse effects on plasma cortisol, PGE_2, and IFN-γ levels.

3.6.3 Lipid Peroxides

In the past decade, research evidence has accumulated that strenuous aerobic exercise is associated with oxidative stress and tissue damage. There is an indication that the generation of oxygen free radicals and other reactive oxygen species may be the underlying mechanism for exercise-induced oxidative damage, but a causal relationship remains to be established. Depletion of each of the antioxidant systems increases the vulnerability of various tissues and cellular components to reactive oxygen species. Because acute strenuous exercise and chronic exercise training increase the oxidative stress and thus the consumption of various antioxidants, it is conceivable that dietary supplementation of specific antioxidants would be beneficial.[124] During severe oxidative stress such as strenuous exercise, the enzymatic and nonenzymatic antioxidant systems of skeletal muscle are not able to cope with the massive free-radical formation, which results in an increase in lipid peroxidation. However, exercise and training appear to augment the body's antioxidant defense system.[125]

Whether this augmented defense system can keep up with the increase in lipid peroxidation with exercise is not known. Vitamin E decreases exercise-induced lipid peroxidation. The exercise may increase superoxide anion generation in the heart, and the increase in the activity of superoxide dismutase (SOD) in skeletal muscle may be indirect evidence for exercise-induced superoxide formation. Therefore, administration of SOD may prevent exercise-induced oxidative stress. Antioxidant enzymes play an important role in defending the cells against free-radical-mediated oxidative damage. An acute bout of exercise can increase activity of certain antioxidant enzymes in various tissues. The mechanism of this activation is unclear. Exercise training has little effect on hepatic or myocardial enzyme systems but can cause adaptive responses in skeletal muscle antioxidant enzymes, particularly glutathione peroxidase.

A growing amount of evidence indicates that free radicals play an important role as mediators of skeletal-muscle damage and inflammation after strenuous exercise. It has been postulated that the generation of oxygen free radicals is increased during exercise as a result of increases in mitochondrial oxygen consumption and electron transport flux, inducing lipid peroxidation.[126] Trained individuals have an advantage over untrained, as training results in increased activity of several major antioxidant enzymes and overall antioxdiant status.

The plasma lipid peroxides level ranged from 0.19–1.65 nmoles/ml at rest and increased to 5.80–12.35 nmoles/ml after an exhaustive endurance run.[122] The plasma lipid peroxides were higher after the endurance run in both men and women. Plasma lipid peroxide concentration was lower on the high-fat diet than on the lower-fat diets. When data were analyzed to determine the effects of the fat intake level and endurance run in women, the plasma lipid peroxide level was found to be lower on the high-fat diet than on the lower-fat diets after exercise.

3.7 CONCLUSIONS/FUTURE DIRECTIONS

It is important that athletes involved in intensive training receive nutritionally correct and well balanced diets. In addition, it is important to keep competitive athletes healthy. Although we have made progress in these areas in the last decade,

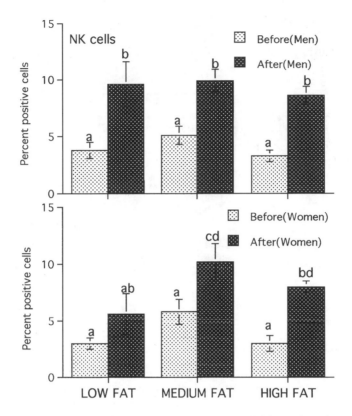

Figure 3.3 Effects of exercise (VO$_{2\,max}$) and level of dietary lipids on the number of natural killer cells in peripheral blood mononuclear cells of endurance trained runners (resting level and after VO$_{2max}$ test). Values are mean ± SEM of 7 subjects per group. Exercise significantly increased the number of NK cells (at $P < 0.0001$); Diet effect $P < 0.01$ (LF vs.. MF $P < 0.001$; MF vs. HF at $P < 0.01$) as revealed by Fisher's PLSD test. Values without a common letter are significantly different at $P < 0.05$.

many questions remain unanswered. As intensive training can be very demanding, all athletes need a sufficient number of calories to meet their energy requirements.

The sources of these calories (fat, carbohydrate, and protein) should meet their expenditure during training and performance. Failure to accomplish this results in depletion of intramuscular stores of glycogen and fats and reduces performance. It is clear that diets with less than 20% carbohydrates or 20% fats are insufficient to maintain intramuscular stores of glycogen and fats, respectively. Increasing carbohydrates on a low-carbohydrate diet and fats on a low-fat diet improve exercise performance. The optimum blend of fats and carbohydrates for different athletes is controversial, and remains to be investigated. Fat intake may be particularly important in female athletes where low-caloric/fat intake diets are associated with amenorrhea, as well as diminished exercise performance.

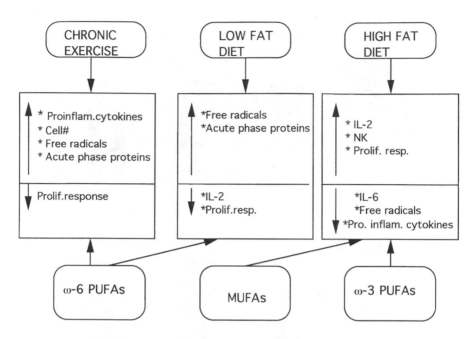

Figure 3.4: Summary of how dietary lipids may modulate the exercise-induced effects on the immune system.

There is a perception that athletes are susceptible to infectious illness, increased oxidative stress, and delayed muscle repair, implying impaired immune function (see Figure 3.4). This is not universally found and may, in fact, be true only in athletes who are overtrained or participate in competitions too frequently. A confounding variable that affects the immune system in overtrained athletes is their low caloric/fat intake. In addition to the low intramuscular stores, it has been shown that low-calorie and low-fat diets do not provide enough essential micronutrients, which may compromise the immune system. Thus, increasing fat intake might provoke adaptive responses and prevent the detrimental effects on exercise performance. The data presented above support the conclusion that running training up to 40 miles/week and a diet comprising 42% fat did not compromise the immune system.

However, a low-fat diet comprising too few calories is immune suppressive in runners (Figure 3.4). The type and quantity of dietary fat (See Figure 3.3), when appropriately selected, may have potential in partially overcoming some of the transitory proinflammatory immunosuppressive effects of exercise. Thus, it may be possible to overcome some of the adverse immune-suppressive effects of exercise on the immune system of runners through carefully selecting both the quantity and type of dietary fat. As lipids are powerful mediators of the immune system, and they are known to exert their effects on cytokines, hormones, etc., the immunosuppressive effects of strenuous exercise could be corrected by carefully selecting the dietary lipids. Consuming increasing levels of dietary fat, up to 42% of total caloric intake, does not elevate fasting levels of TG, total cholesterol, or HDL cholesterol in the plasma of runners, suggesting that higher fat consumption can be recommended for athletes without increasing the risk of cardiovascular disease.

Further studies in this area are needed to address the effects of the total calories taken in as fat and the types and amounts of fats that are protective to the immune system in different types of athletes. The intensity and duration of exercise will affect both carbohydrate and fat oxidation and thus determine the amount of carbohydrates and the amounts and types of fat that should be ingested to meet the demands of the exercise and maintain immunocompetence.

High-fat diets are suggested to increase FFA availability and spare muscle glycogen, resulting in improved performance. High-fat diets may provoke adaptive responses, preventing the detrimental effects to exercise performance. Further studies in this area are needed to address the effects of the types of fat, type of calories with endurance, performance, and other type and intensities of exercise on immune status and hormone status of athletes.

Taken together, the results presented above suggest that it may be possible to overcome some of the adverse immune-suppressive effects of exercise on the immune system of athletes through carefully selecting both quantity and type of dietary fat. Consuming increasing levels of dietary fat, up to 40%, does not elevate fasting levels of TGs, total cholesterol, or HDL cholesterol in plasma in these subjects, suggesting high fat consumption can be recommended for marathon runners and athletes who are undergoing intensive training. The upper limit of fat intake and lower limits of carbohydrate intake are still not known. As lipids are powerful mediators of the immune system, and they are known to exert their effects on cytokines, hormones, etc., the immunosuppressive effects of strenuous exercise could be corrected by carefully selecting the dietary lipids.

ACKNOWLEDGMENTS

The authors wish to thank Dr. Nadine Fisher, assistant professor, Department of Occupational Therapy and the Rehabilitation Sciences Program, SUNY at Buffalo, for reading the manuscript and for her valuable suggestions.

REFERENCES

1. Brooks, G.A., Importance of the "crossover" concept in exercise metabolism, *Clin. Exer. Pharm. Physiol.*, 24, 889, 1997.
2. Muoio, D.M., Leddy, J.J., Horvath, P.J., Awad, A.B., and Pendergast, D.R., Effect of dietary fat on metabolic adjustments to maximal VO_2 and endurance in runners, *Med. Sci. Sports. Exerc.*, 26, 81, 1994.
3. Lambert, E.V., Speechly, D.P., Dennis, S.C., and Noakes, T.D., Enhanced endurance in trained cyclists during moderate intensity exercise following 2 weeks adaptation to a high fat diet, *Eur. J. Appl. Physiol.*, 69, 287, 1994.
4. Pendergast, D.P., Horvath, P.J., Leddy, J.J., and Venkatraman, J.T., The role of dietary fat on performance, metabolism, and health, *Amer. J. Sports Med.*, 24, S53, 1996.

5. Thompson, J.L., Manore, M.M., Skinner, J.S., Ravussin, E., and Spraul, M., Daily energy expenditure in male endurance athletes with differing energy intakes, *Med. Sci. Sports Exerc.,* 27, 347, 1995.

6. Jeukendrup, A.E. and Saris, W.H.M., Fat as a fuel during exercise, in *Nutrition for Sport and Exercise,* 2nd ed., Berning, J.R., Nelson-Steen, S., Eds., Aspen Publishers Inc., Gaithersburg, Maryland, 59, 1998.

7. Wolfe, R.R., Klein, S., Carraro, F., and Weber, J-M., Role of triglyceride–fatty acid cycle in controlling fat metabolism in humans during and after exercise, *Am. J. Physiol.,* 258, E382, 1990.

8. Romijn, J.A., Coyle, E.F., Sidossis, L.S., Gastaldelli, A., Horowitz, J.F., Endert, E., and Wolfe, R.R., Regulation of endogenous fat and carbohydrate metabolism in relation to exercise intensity and duration, *Am. J. Physiol.,* 265, E380, 1993.

9. Havel, R.J., Pernow, B., and Jones, N.L., Uptake and release of free fatty acids and other metabolites in the legs of exercising men, *J. Appl. Physiol.,* 23, 90, 1967.

10. Roberts, T.J., Weber, J.M., Hoppeler, H., Weibel, E.R., and Taylor, C.R., Design of the oxygen and substrate pathways: II. Defining the upper limit of carbohydrate and fat oxidation, *J. Exp. Biol.,* 199, 1651, 1996.

11. Vock, R., Hoppeler, H., Claassen, H., Wu, D.X.Y., Billeter, R., Weber, J.M., Taylor, C.R., and Weibel, E.R., Design of the oxygen and substrate pathways: VI Structural basis of intracellular substrate supply to mitochondria in muscle cells, *J. Exp. Biol.,* 199, 1689, 1996.

12. Holloszy, J.O. and Coyle, E.F., Adaptations of skeletal muscle to endurance exercise and their metabolic consequences, *J. Appl. Physiol.: Resp. Env. Excer. Phys.,* 56, 831, 1984.

13. Coggan, A.R. and Williams, B.D., Metabolic adaptations to endurance training: substrate metabolism during exercise, *Exercise Metabolism,* Hargreaves, M., Ed., Human Kinetics Publishers, Champaign, IL, 41, 1995.

14. Starling, R.D., Trappe, T.A., Parcell, A.C., Kerr, C.G., Fink, W.J., and Costill, D.L., Effects of diet on muscle triglyceride and endurance performance, *J. Appl. Physiol.,* 82, 1185, 1997.

15. Coyle, E.F., Coggan, A.R., Hemmert, M.K., and Ivy, J.L., Muscle glycogen utilization during prolonged strenuous exercise when fed carbohydrate, *J. Appl. Physiol.* 61, 165, 1986.

16. Horvath, P.J., Eagan, C.K., Leddy, J.J., and Pendergast, D.R., Effect of dietary fat level on performance and metabolism in trained male and female runners (abstract), *FASEB J.,* 10, 1658, 1996.

17. Venkatraman, J.T., Rowland, J.A., Denardin, E., Horvath, P.J., and Pendergast, D.R., Influence of the level of dietary lipid intake and maximal exercise on the immune status in runners, *J. Med. Sci. Sports Exerc.,* 29, 333, 1997.

18. Blair, S.N., Ellsworth, N.M., Haskell, W.L., Stern, M.P., Farquhar, J.W., and Wood, P.D., Comparison of nutrient intake in middle-aged men and women runners and controls, *Med. Sci. Sports. Exerc.,* 13, 310,1981.

19. Vallieres, F., Tremblay, A., and St-Jean L., Study of the energy balance and the nutritional status of highly trained female swimmers, *Nutr. Res.,* 9, 699, 1989.

20. Benson, J., Gillien, D.M., Bourdet, K., and Lossli, A.R., Inadequate nutrition and chronic calorie restriction in adolescent ballerinas, *Physician Sports Med.,* 79, October, 1985.

21. Nieman, D.C., Butler, J.V., Pollett, L.M., Dietrich, S.J., and Lutz, R.D., Nutrient intake of marathon runners, *J. Am. Dietet. Assoc.,* 89, 1273, 1989.

22. Chen, J.D., Wang, J.F., Li, K.J., Zhao, Y.W., Wang, S.W., Jiao, Y., and Hou, X.Y., Nutritional problems and measures in elite and amateur athletes, *Am. J. Clin. Nutr.,* 49, 1084, 1989.

23. Mulligan, K. and Butterfield, G.E., Discrepancies between energy intake and expenditure in physically active women, *Brit. J. Nutr.,* 64, 23,1990.

24. Tuschl, R.J., Platte, P., Laessle, R.G., Sticher, W., and Pirke, K.M., Energy expenditure and everyday eating behavior in health young women, *Am. J. Clin. Nutr.,* 52, 81, 1990.

25. Packer, L., Protective role of vitamin E in biological systems, *Am. J. Clin. Nutr.,* 53, 1050S, 1991.

26. Moffatt, R.J., Dietary status of elite female high school gymnasts: inadequacy of vitamin and mineral intake, *J. Am. Dietet. Assoc.,* 84, 1361,1984.

27. Grandjean, A.C., Macronutrient intake of US athletes compared with the general population and recommendations made for athletes, *Am. J. Clin. Nutr.,* 49, 1070, 1989.

28. Short, S.H., and Short, W.R., Four-year study of university athletes' dietary intake, *J. Am. Dietet. Assoc.,* 82, 632, 1983.

29. Hickson, J.F. Jr., Duke, M.A., Risser, W.L., Johnson, C.W., Palmer, R., and Stockton, J.E., Nutritional intake from food sources of high school football athletes, *J. Am. Dietet. Assoc.,* 87, 1656, 1987

30. Welch, P.K., Zager, K.D., Endres, J., and Poon, S.W., Nutrition education, body composition, and dietary intake of female college athletes, *Phys. Sports Med.,* 63, January, 1987.

31. Strauzenberg, S.E., Schneider, F.. Donath, R., Zerbes, H., and Kohler, E., The problem of dieting in training and athletic performance., *Bibliotheca Nutrition et Dieta.,* 27, 133, 1979.

32. Steel, J.E., A nutritional study of Australian Olympic athletes, *Med. J. Austr.,* 2, 119, 1970.

33. Ready, A.E., Nutrient intake of the Canadian women's Olympic field hockey team, *Can. Home Econ. J.,* 37, 29, 1987.

34. Hickson, J.F., Wolinsky, I., Pivarnik, J.M., Neuman, E.A., Itak, J.F., and Stockton, J.E., Nutritional profile of football athletes eating from a training table, *Nutr. Res.* 7, 27, 1987b.

35. Ellsworth, N.M., Hewett, B.F., and Haskell, W.L., Nutrient intake of elite male and female Nordic skiers, *Phys Sports Med.,* 78, February,1985.

36. deWijn, J.F., Leusink, J., and Post, G.B., Diet, body composition, and physical condition of champion rowers during periods of training and out of training, *Bibl. Nutr. Diet.,* 27, 143, 1979.

37. Manore, M.M., Besenfelder, P.D., Wells, C.L., Carroll, S.S., and Hooker, S.P., Nutrient intakes and iron status in female long-distance runners during training, *J. Am. Dietet. Assoc.,* 89, 257, 1989.

38. Lally, D.A., Wang, J.H., Goebert, D.A., Quigley, R.D., and Hartung, G.H., Performance, training, and dietary characteristics of American and Japanese wheelchair marathoners, *Med. Sci. Sports Exerc.,* 23, S101, 1991.

39. Deuster, P.A., Kyle, S.B., Moser, P.B., Vigersky, R.A., Singh, A., and Schoomaker, E.B., Nutritional survey of highly trained women runners, *Am. J. Clin. Nutr.,* 44, 954, 1986.

40. Rico-Sanz, J., Frontera, W.R., Mole, P.A., Rivera-Brown, A., Meredith, C.N., Dietary and performance assessment of elite soccer players during a period of intense training, *Int. J. Sports Nutr.* 8, 230, 1998.

41. Berning, J., Swimmers' nutrition knowledge and practice, *Sports Nutr. News,* 4, 1, 1986.
42. Worme, J.D., Doubt, T.J., Singh, A., Ryan, C.J., Moses, F.M., and Deuster, P.A., Dietary patterns, gastrointestinal complaints, and nutrition knowledge of recreational triathletes, *Am. J. Clin. Nutr.,* 51, 690. 1990.
43. Burke, L.M., and Read, R.S.D., Diet patterns of elite Australian male triathletes, *Phys. Sports Med.,* 140, February, 1987.
44. Bazzarre, T.L., Kleiner, S.M., and Litchford, M.D., Nutrient intake, body fat, and lipid profiles of competitive male and female bodybuilders, *J. Am.Coll. Nutr.,* 9, 136, 1990.
45. Shultz, T.D., Wilcox, R.B., Spuehler, J.M., and Howie, B.J., Dietary and hormonal interrelationships in premenopausal women: evidence for a relationship between dietary nutrients and plasma prolactin levels, *Am. J. Clin. Nutr.,* 46, 905, 1987.
46. Goldin, B.R., Adlercreutz, H., Gorbach, S.L., Warram, J.H., Dwyer, J.T., Swenson, L., and Woods, M.N., Estrogen excretion patterns and plasma levels in vegetarian and omnivorous women, *New Eng. J. Med.,* 307, 1542, 1982.
47. Myerson, M., Gutin, B., Warren, M.P., May, M.T., Contento, I., Lee, M., Pi-Sunyer, F.X., Pierson, R.N., and Brooks-Gunn, J., Resting metabolic rate and energy balance in amenorrheic and eumennorrheic runners, *Med. Sci. Sports Exerc.,* 23, 15, 1991.
48. Baer, J.T. and Taper, L.J., Amenorrheic and eumenorrheic adolescent runners: dietary intake and exercise training status, *J. Am. Dietet. Assoc.,* 92, 89, 1992.
49. Grundy, S.M., Multifactorial etiology of hypercholesterolemia: implications for prevention of coronary heart disease, *Arterioscler. Thromb.,* 11, 1619, 1991.
50. Grundy, S.M., Cholesterol and coronary disease: future directions, *J. Am. Med. Assoc.,* 264, 3053.
51. Parthasarathy, S., Khoo, J.C., Miller, E., Barnett, J., Witztum, J.L., and Steinberg, D., Low-density lipoprotein rich in oleic acid is protected against oxidative modification: implications for dietary prevention of atherosclerosis, *Proc. Natl. Acad. Sci.,* 87, 3894, 1990.
52. Weymen, C., Belin, J., Smith, A.D., and Thompson, R.H., Linoleic acid as an immunosuppressive agent, *Lancet,* 2, 33, 1975.
53. Kris-Etherton, P.M., Krummel, D., Russell, M.E., Dreon, D., Mackey, S., Borcher, J., and Wood, P.D., The effect of diet on plasma lipids, lipoproteins, and coronary heart disease, *J. Amer. Dietet. Assoc.,* 88, 1373, 1988.
54. Hunt, J.N. and Knox, M.T., Regulation of gastric emptying, in *Handbook of Physiology, Sec. 6 Vol.4, Am. Physiol. Soc.,* Bethesda, MD, 1968, 1917.
55. Simi, B., Sempore, B., Mayet, M.H., and Favier, R.J., Additive effects of training and high-fat diet on energy metabolism during exercise, *J. Appl. Physiol.,* 71, 197, 1991.
56. Keast, D., Cameron, K., and Morton, A.R., Exercise and immune response, *Sports Med.,* 5, 248, 1988.
57. Nieman, D.C. and Nehlsen-Cannarella, S.L., The immune response to exercise. *Semin. Hematology,* 31, 166, 1994.
58. Nieman, D.C., Immune response to heavy exertion, *J. Appl. Physiol.,* 82, 1385, 1997.
59. Nieman, D.C., Upper respiratory tract infections and exercise, *Thorax,* 50, 1229, 1995.
60. Pedersen, B.K., and Bruunsgaard, H., How physical exercise influences the establishment of infections, *Sports Med.,* 19, 393, 1995.
61. Mackinnon, L.T., *Exercise and Immunology: Current Issues in Exercise Science Series,* (Monograph number 2), Champaign, IL, Human Kinetics Publishers, 1992, 1.
62. Peters, E.M., Exercise, immunology and upper respiratory tract infections, *Int. J. Sports Med.,* 18, S69-77, 1997.

63. Smith, J.A., Guidelines, standards, and perspectives in exercise immunology, *Med. Sci. Sports Exerc.*, 27, 497, 1995.
64. Nieman, D.C., Johanssen, L.M., and Lee, J.W., Infectious episodes in runners before and after a road race. *J. Sports Med. & Phys. Fitness*, 29, 289, 1989.
65. Kendall, A., Hoffman-Goetz, L., Houston, M., MacNeil, B., and Arumugam, Y., Exercise and blood lymphocyte subset responses: intensity, duration, and subject fitness effects, *J. Applied Physiol.*, 69, 251, 1990.
66. Boas, S.R., Joswiak, M.L., Nixon, P.A., Kurland, G., O'Connor, M.J., Bufalino, K., Orenstein, D.M., and Whiteside, T.L., Effects of anaerobic exercise on the immune system in eight-to seventeen-year-old trained and untrained boys, *J. Pediat.*, 129, 846, 1996.
67. Espersen, G.T., Elbaek, A., Schmidt-Olsen, S., Ejlersen, E., Varming, K., and Grunnet, N., Short-term changes in the immune system of elite swimmers under competition conditions. Different immunomodulation induced by various types of sport, *Scand. J. Med. & Sci. Sports,* 6, 156, 1996.
68. Weiss, C., Kinscherf, R., Roth, S., Friedmann, B., Fischbach, T., Reus, J., Droge, W., and Bartsch, P., Lymphocyte subpopulations and concentrations of soluble CD8 and CD4 antigen after anaerobic training, *Int. J. Sports Med.*, 16, 117, 1995.
69. Espersen, G.T., Elbaek, A., Ernst, E., Toft, E., Kaalund, S., Jersild, C., and Grunnet, N., Effect of physical exercise on cytokines and lymphocyte subpopulations in human peripheral blood, *APMIS*, 98, 395, 1990.
70. Hinton, J.R., Rowbottom, D.G., Keast, D., and Morton, A.R., Acute intensive interval training and *in vitro* t-lymphocyte function, *Int. J. Sports Med.*, 18, 130, 1997.
71. LaPerriere, A., Antoni, M.H., Ironson, G., Perry, A., McCabe, P., Klimas, N., Helder, L., Schneiderman, N., and Fletcher, M.A., Effects of aerobic exercise training on lymphocyte subpopulations, *Int. J. Sports Med.*, 15 Suppl 3, S127, 1994.
72. Smith, J., Chi, D., Salazar, S., Krish, G., Berk, S., Reynolds, S., and Cambron, G., Effect of moderate exercise on proliferative responses of peripheral blood mononuclear cells, *J. Sports Med. & Phys. Fitness,* 33, 152, 1993.
73. Gabriel, H., Kullmer, T., Schwarz, L., Urhausen, A., Weiler, B., Born, P., and Kindermann, W., Circulating leucocyte subpopulations in sedentary subjects following graded maximal exercise with hypoxia, *Eur. J. Appl. Physiol. and Occup. Physiol.*, 67, 348, 1993.
74. Nieman, D.C., Miller, A.R., Henson, D.A., Warren, B.J., Gusewitch, G., Johnson, R.L., Davies, J.M., Butterworth, D.E., and Nehlsen-Cannarella, S.L., Effects of high-vs. moderate exercise-intensity exercise on natural killer cell activity, *Med. Sci Sports & Exerc.,* 25, 1126, 1993.
75. Kawada, E., Kubota, K., Kurabayashi, H., Tamura, K., Tamura, J., and Shirakura, T., Effects of long-term running on lymphocyte subpopulations, *Tohoku J. Exp. Med.,* 167, 273, 1992.
76. Gabriel, H., Urhausen, A., and Kindermann, W., Circulating leucocyte and lymphocyte subpopulations before and after intensive endurance exercise to exhaustion, *Eur. J. Appl. Physiol. & Occup. Physiol.*, 63, 449, 1991.
77. MacNeil, B., Hoffman-Goetz, L., Kendall, A., Houston, M., and Arumugam, Y., Lymphocyte proliferation responses after exercise in men: fitness, intensity, and duration effects, *J. Appl. Physiol.*, 70, 179, 1991.
78. Ferry, A., Picard, F., Duvallet, A., Weill, B., and Rieu, M., Changes in blood leucocyte populations induced by acute maximal and chronic submaximal exercise, *Eur. J. Appl. Physiol. Occup. Physiol.*, 59, 435, 1990.

79. Hoffman-Goetz L., Simpson, J.R., Cipp, N., Arumugam, Y., and Houston, M.E., Lymphocyte subset responses to repeated submaximal exercise in men, *J. Appl. Physiol.*, 68, 1069, 1990.

80. Nieman, D.C., Simandle, S., Henson, D.A., Warren, B.J., Suttles, J., Davis, J.M., Buckley, K.S., Ahle, J.C., Butterworth, D.E., Fagoaga, O.R., and Nehlsen-Cannarella, S.L., Lymphocyte proliferative response to 2.5 h of running, *Int. J. Sports Med.*, 16, 404, 1995.

81. Shinkai, S., Shore, S., Shek, P.N., and Shephard, R.J., Acute exercise and immune function. Relationship between lymphocyte activity and changes in subset counts, *Int. J. Sports Med.*, 13, 452, 1992.

82. Nieman, D.C., Brendle, D., Henson, D.A., Suttles, J., Cook, V.D., Warren, B.J., Butterworth, D.E., Fagoaga, O.R., and Nehlsen-Cannarella, S.L., Immune function in athletes vs.. nonathletes, *Int. J. Sports Med.* 16, 329, 1995.

83. Rivier, A., Pene, J., Chanez, P., Anselme, F., Caillaud, C., Prefaut, C., Godard, P., and Bousquet, J., Release of cytokines by blood monocytes during strenuous exercise, *Int. J. Sports Med.*, 15, 192, 1994.

84. Sprenger, H., Jacobs, C., Nain, M., Gressner, A.M., Prinz, H., Wesemann, W., and Gemsa, D., Enhanced release of cytokines interleukin-2 receptors, and neopterin after long-distance running, *Clin. Immunol. Immunopathol.*, 63, 188, 1992.

85. Cannon, J.G., Meydani, S.N., Fielding, R.A., Fiatarone, M.A., Meydani, M., Farhangmehr, M., Orencole, S.F., Blumberg, J.B., and Evans, W.J., Acute phase response in exercise. II. Associations between vitamin E, cytokines, and muscle proteolysis, *Am. J. Physiol.*, 260, R1235, 1991.

86. Cashmore, G.C., Davies, C.T., and Few, J.D., Relationship between increase in plasma cortisol concentration and rate of cortisol secretion during exercise in man, *J. Endocrinol.*, 72, 109, 1977.

87. Marinelli, M., Roi, G.S., Giacometti, M., Bonini, P., and Banfi, G., Cortisol, testosterone and free testosterone in athletes performing a marathon at 4000m altitude, *Hormone Res.*, 41, 225, 1994.

88. McCarthy, D.A., and Dale, M.M., The leucocytosis of exercise. A review and model, *Sports Med.*, 6, 333, 1988.

89. Hoffmann-Goetz, L.,and Pedersen, B.K., Exercise and the immune system: a model of the stress response?, *Immunol. Today*, 15, 382, 1994.

90. Kjaer, M., Epinephrine and some other hormonal responses to exercise in man: with special reference to physical training, *Int. J. Sports Med.*,10, 2, 1989.

91. Perna, F.M., and Mcdowell, S.L., Role of psychological stress in cortisol recovery from exhaustive exercise among elite athletes, *Int. J. Behav. Med.*, 2, 13, 1995.

92. Davies, C.T., and Few, J.D., Effects of exercise on adrenocortical function, *J. Appl. Physiol.*, 35, 887, 1973.

93. Silverman, H.G., and Mazzeo, R.S., Hormonal responses to maximal and submaximal exercise in trained and untrained men of various ages, *J. Gerontol.*, 51, B30, 1996.

94. Tilz, G.P., Domej, W., Diez-Ruiz, A., Weiss, G., Brezinschek, R., Brezinschek, H.P., Huttl, E., Pristautz, H., Wachter, H., and Fuchs, D., Increased immune activation during and after physical exercise, *Immunobiol.*, 188, 194, 1993.

95. Fernandes, G., Effect of dietary fish oil supplement on autoimmune disease: changes in lymphoid cell subsets, oncogene mRNA expression and neuroendocrine hormones, in *Health Effects of Fish and Fish Oil,* Chandra, R.K., Ed., ARTS Biomedical Publications, St. John's, Newfoundland, 409, 1989.

96. Johnston, P.V., Lipid modulation of immune responses, in *Nutrition and Immunology, Contemporary Issues in Clinical Nutrition,* Vol.II, Chandra, R.K., Ed., Alan R. Liss, Inc., New York, 1988, 37.

97. Peck, M.D., Interactions of lipids with immune function II. Experimental and clinical studies of lipids and immunity, *J. Nutr. Biochem.,* 5, 514, 1994.

98. Fernandes, G., Bysani, C., Venkatraman, J.T., Tomar, V., and Zhao, W., Increased TGFb and decreased oncogene expression by ω–3 fatty acids in the spleen delays onset of autoimmune disease in B/W mice, *J. Immunol.,*152, 5979, 1994.

99. Endres, S., Ghorbani,R., Kelley, V.E., Georgilis, K., Lonnemann, G., van der Meer, J.W., Cannon, J.G., Rogers, T, S., Klempner, M.S., Weber, P.C., et al. The effect of dietary supplementation with *n*-3 polyunsaturated fatty acids on the synthesis of interleukin-1 and tumor necrosis factor by mononuclear cells, *New Eng. J. Med.,* 320, 265, 1989.

100. Venkatraman, J.T., Immunomodulatory effects of ω–3 lipids and vitamin E on proliferative response, lymphoid subsets and *in vitro* production of cytokines by splenocytes in autoimmune-prone MRL/*lpr* mice, *FASEB J.,* 12, A870, Abst #5038, 1998.

101. Fernandes, G. and Venkatraman, J.T., Role of omega-3 fatty acids in health and disease, *Nutr. Res.,*13 (Suppl), S19, 1993.

102. Fernandes, G., Venkatraman, J.T., Khare, A., Horbach, G.J.M.J., and Friedrichs, W., Modulation of gene expression in autoimmune disease by food restriction and dietary lipids, *Proc. Soc. Exp. Biol. Med.,* 193, 16, 1990.

103. Venkatraman, J.T., Chandrasekar, B., Kim, J.D., and Fernandes, G., Effect of *n*-3 and *n*-6 fatty acids on activities and expression of hepatic antioxidant enzymes in autoimmune-prone NZB/NZWF1 mice, *Lipids,* 29, 561, 1994.

104. Banerjee, N. and Rosenthal, M.D., High-affinity incorporation of 20-carbon polyunsaturated fatty acids by human skin fibroblasts, *Biochim. Biophys. Acta,* 835, 533, 1985.

105. Iritani, N., Ikeda, Y., and Fukuda, H., Physiological impairment in linoleic acid deficiency of rats and the effect of n-3 polyunsaturated fatty acids, *J. Nutr. Sci. & Vitaminol.,* 30, 179, 1984.

106. Souba, W.W., Cytokine control of nutrition and metabolism in critical illness, *Curr. Problems in Surg.,* 31, 577, 1994.

107. Konig, D., Berg, A., Weinstock, C., Keul, J., and Northoff, H., Essential fatty acids, immune function, and exercise, *Exerc. Immunol. Rev.,* 3, 1, 1997.

108. Grunfeld, C. and Feingold, K.R., Regulation of lipid metabolism by cytokines during host defense, *Nutrition,* 12 (1 Suppl), S24 1996.

109. Stouthard, J.M., Romijn, J.A., Van der Poll, T., Endert, E., Klein, S., Bakker, P.J., Veenhof, C.H., and Sauerwein, H.P., Endocrinologic and metabolic effects of interleukin-6 in humans, *Amer. J. Physiol.,* 268 (5 Pt 1), E813, 1995.

110. Espat, N.J., Moldawer, L.L., and Copeland, E.M. 3rd., Cytokine-mediated alterations in host metabolism prevent nutritional repletion in cachectic cancer patients, *J. Surg. Oncol.,* 58, 77, 1995.

111. Santoli, D, and Zurier, R.B., Prostaglandin E precursor fatty acids inhibit human IL-2 production by a prostaglandin E-dependent mechanism, *Immunology,* 143, 1303, 1989.

112. Meydani, S.N., Lichenstein, A.H., Cornwall, S., Meydani, M., Goldin, B.R., Rasmussen, H., Dinarello, C.A., and Schaefer, E.J., Immunologic effects of national cholesterol education panel step-2 diets with and without fish-derived n-3 fatty acid enrichment, *J. Clin. Invest.,* 92, 105, 1993.

113. Virella, G., Kilpatrick, J.M., Rugeles, M.T., Hyman, B., and Russell R. Depression of humoral responses and phagocytic functions *in vivo* and *in vitro* by fish oil and eicosapentaenoic acid, *Clin. Immunol. Immunopathol.,* 52: 257, 1989.

114. Gemsa, D., Leser, H.G., Deimann, W., and Resch, K., Suppression of T lymphocyte proliferation during lymphoma growth in mice: role of PGE_2-producing lymphocyte proliferation, suppressor macrophages, *Immunobiol.*, 161, 385, 1982.

115. Tvede, N., Kappel, M., Halkjar-Kristensen, J., Galbo, H., Pedersen, B.K., The effect of light, moderate and severe exercise on lymphocyte subsets, natural and lymphokine activated killer cells, lymphocyte proliferative response and interleukin–2 production, *Int. J. Sports Med.,* 14, 275, 1993.

116. Pedersen, B.K., Tvede, N., Klarlund, K., Christensen, L.D., Hansen, F.R., Galbo, H., Kharazmi, A., and Halkjaer-Kristensen. J., Indomethacin *in vitro* and *in vivo* abolishes post-exercise suppression of natural killer cell activity in peripheral blood, *Int. J. Sports Med.,* 11, 127, 1990.

117. Smith, L.L., Wells, J.M., Houmard, J.A., Smith, S.T., Israel, R.G., Chenier, T.C., and Pennington, S.N., Increases in plasma prostaglandin E_2 after eccentric exercise, a preliminary report, *Hor. Metab. Res.*, 25, 451, 1993.

118. Ogle, C.K., Tchervenkov, J., Alexander, J.W., Ogle, J.D., Palkert, D., Taylor, A., Barnwell, S., and Warden, G.D., The effect of high lipid diet on *in vitro* prostaglandin E_2 and thromboxane B_2 production by splenic macrophages, *J. Paren. Ent. Nutr.*,14, 250, 1990.

119. Miller, W.C., Bryce, G.R., and Conlee, R.K., Adaptations to a high-fat diet that increase exercise endurance in male rats, *J. Appl. Physiol., Resp. Env. Exerc. Phys.,* 56, 78, 1984.

120. Phinney, S.D., Bistrian, B.R., Evans, W.J., Grevino, E., and Blackburn, G.L., The human metabolic response to chronic ketosis without caloric restriction: preservation of submaximal exercise capability with reduced carbohydrate oxidation, *Metabolism: Clinic. Exp.*, 32, 769, 1983.

121. Venkatraman, J.T. and Pendergast, D., Effects of the level of dietary fat intake and endurance exercise on plasma cytokines in runners, *Med. Sci. Sports Exerc.,* 30, 1198, 1998.

122. Feng, X., Pendergast, D.R., and Venkatraman, J.T., Effects of dietary fat on plasma hormones in runners, *FASEB J.,* 11, A580, Ab#3357, 1997.

123. Venkatraman, J.T. and Pendergast, D.R., Effect of dietary lipids and exercise on cellular immune responses and plasma cytokines and hormones in runners. (Abstract) *Int. Soc. Exerc. Immunol. Symposium, May-21–23,1999,* Rome, Italy.

124. Ji, L.L., Exercise and oxidative stress: role of cellular antioxidant systems, *Exerc. Sports Rev.,* 23, 135, 1995.

125. Clarkson, P.M., Micronutrients and exercise: anti-oxidants and minerals, *J. Sports Sci.*, 13, S11, 1995.

126. Dekkers, J.C., van Doornen, L.J., and Kemper, H.C., The role of antioxidant vitamins and enzymes in the prevention of exercise-induced muscle damage, *Sports Med.,* 21, 213, 1996.

CHAPTER 4

Protein, Exercise, and Immunity

David G. Rowbottom

CONTENTS

4.1 INTRODUCTION

Malnutrition is widely recognized as a potential source of increased morbidity and mortality throughout the world. In many cases, it is not simply insufficient dietary intake of energy, but more specifically a shortage of dietary protein, leading to what has become known as protein-energy malnutrition. In recent years, our understanding of this interaction has grown to include an appreciation of the essential role of dietary protein for the optimal functioning of the immune system. In fact, protein-energy malnutrition is now considered one of the most common causes of immunodeficiency and immune dysfunction throughout the world.[1] An insufficiency of dietary protein is not a condition restricted to children in the developing world, although this is clearly where its prevalence is most noticeable. Cases of protein-energy malnutrition in the developed world are widely reported in populations such as hospitalized patients,[2, 3] the elderly,[4] and sometimes in anorexia nervosa.[5] In these individuals, where the protein requirements of the body are not being met by dietary intake, a clear link has been established between this lack of protein availability and an impaired immune response.

Athletes, and particularly those who engage in extensive and/or intensive training programs, have been widely reported to have an increased rate of protein turnover.[6] Consequently, these athletes have an increased requirement for dietary protein intake to meet this need. A failure to nutritionally meet this level of protein turnover will lead to a net protein deficiency, which has the potential to expose the athlete to an immunodeficient state. Anecdotal and epidemiological evidence has associated athletes undertaking intensive and extensive training with increased rates of infection and potentially impaired immune function.[7-9] The central question this chapter will attempt to explore is whether there is any association between exercise-induced immunosuppression, and a net protein deficiency through a combination of high protein turnover and inadequate nutritional intake of protein.

4.2 PROTEIN AND IMMUNE FUNCTION

The essential role of dietary protein for optimal immune function was highlighted by early classical studies.[10] Healthy adults were fed a diet containing either 0.1, 1.0 or 2.0 g protein/kg body weight each day for a period of 10 weeks. At the end of the study period, those receiving the lowest daily amount of protein had an impaired antibody response to tetanus antigen.

It is not essentially surprising that host defense mechanisms are impaired during periods of dietary protein inadequacy. Many processes of immune development (such as the maturation of stem cells) and proliferation (such as the response of T-lymphocytes to antigen) require the synthesis of new protein. Additionally, the complex interactions among the different aspects of the immune response are regulated by a series of cytokines, complement and immunoglobulins — chemical messengers all of which require *de novo* protein synthesis. Protein malnutrition is likely to result in an inavailability of essential amino acid precursors, impaired RNA and protein synthesis, and consequently an impaired immune response. Although there are many interrelated aspects to a healthy immune response, it has been reported that cell-mediated immunity in particular is most affected by protein deficiencies. Common observations in protein-energy malnutrition have included atrophy of lymphoid organs, a reduction in circulating leucocytes — T-lymphocytes in particular —

depressed lymphocyte proliferative responses, and cutaneous delayed hypersensitivity reactions.[11–14]

Unfortunately, there is very little direct evidence for an effect of protein deficiency or even protein supplementation on the immune function of athletes. The important question that needs clarification is not whether immunosuppressive effects occur, since there is ample evidence for an effect of dietary protein inadequacy on immune function (Table 1). Rather, protein-energy malnutrition is not a discrete entity, but may be represented as a spectrum of malnourished states from the severe to the mild. The area that needs clarification, and is most crucial in applying information to the athletic population, is whether the immunosuppressive effects occur at all levels of protein deficiency, or if a threshold level exists below which immunosuppression is observed.

Many studies have used serum concentrations of albumin as a quantitative indicator of the degree of malnutrition.[2,3] The rationale has been that those proteins with a rapid turnover may be useful for indicating current protein status and turnover.[15] Several authors have shown that serum albumin can accurately reflect body protein stores and that albumin synthesis by the liver is a sensitive index of dietary protein intake.[16] For the purposes of this chapter, serum albumin concentrations will be used to indicate protein status. The associations between serum albumin status and immune function will be reviewed in protein-energy malnutrition, with a view to identifying a potential threshold level below which immune function can be observed to be impaired. This will then be used as a means of relating potential negative effect in athletes, where serum albumin concentrations have been reported.

Table 4.1   **Summary of the Effects of Protein-Energy Malnutrition on Cell-Mediated Immunity Reported in Malnourished Children, Hospitalized Patients, the Elderly and Individuals with Anorexia Nervosa.**

Immune Parameter		Reference
↓ cutaneous delayed hypersensitivity reaction		2, 5, 13, 20, 21, 24
Circulating cell numbers:	↓ leucocytes	5
	↓ lymphocytes	24, 26
	↓ T-lymphocytes	1, 24, 26
	↓ T-helper lymphocytes	1, 5, 24
	↓ T-suppressor lymphocytes	1, 24, 26
Cell function tests:	↓ lymphocyte proliferation	5, 21, 24, 26
	↓ natural-killer-cell cytotoxicity	17, 18

4.2.1   Malnourished Children

The prevalence of malnutrition in children in developing countries is well known. The World Health Organization (WHO) recommends a minimum protein intake of 0.8 g/kg body weight/day for the needs of a sedentary individual. Although the actual level of protein intake has rarely been quantified in studies of malnourished children, indirect evidence is usually apparent in terms of symptoms of marasmus (underweight) or kwashiorkor (edema). A consistent finding has been that those children with protein-energy malnutrition have impaired cutaneous delayed hypersensitivity reactions[13] as well as other evidence of impaired cell-mediated immunity. Thymic atrophy, lymphoid tissue atrophy and lymphocytopenia, with particular reductions in circulating numbers of T-helper lymphocytes and natural-killer cells, are commonly observed in malnourished children.[11] While T-lymphocyte proliferation responses to mitogen are also reduced, the use of autologous serum has been shown to produce even greater deficiencies,[1] suggesting that serum factors may be impaired in addition to cellular mechanisms. Depressed natural-killer-cell activity, as assessed by cytotoxicity against ^{51}Cr-labelled K562 cells, has also been reported in children with protein-energy malnutrition.[17,18] Specific lytic activity was as low as 2.5% using a 25:1 effector to target ratio. This compares with values of 32% reported in healthy adults in the United States using a 20:1 ratio.[19]

The essential task for the application of this information is to relate the immune-function impairments to reported levels of protein status. In a recent study, malnourished children were graded on the basis of weight for age and symptoms of kwashiorkor.[12] Normal-weight children (>80% of weight for age) and underweight children (60–80% weight for age) were not significantly different in terms of serum protein (69.7 ± 5.9 vs. 67.5 ± 7.2 g/l) or serum albumin (42.8 ± 3.2 vs. 40.4 ± 7.2 g/l) concentrations and were also not significantly different in a number of immune parameters. Those children classified as either marasmus (<60% weight for age) or marasmus kwashiorkor (<60% weight for age and symptoms of edema) had significantly lower serum protein (55.2 ± 12.5 and 53.0 ± 10.0 g/l) and serum albumin (29.0 ± 8.6 and 27.5 ± 5.7 g/l) concentrations than the normal-weight children. These latter two groups also had significantly lower serum complement C3 concentrations, which may be indicative of a reduced protein availability in these populations. Unfortunately, lymphocyte subpopulations were expressed as percentages and not absolute numbers of circulating cells, making any meaningful comparison of cell-mediated-immunity status difficult. Taken together, these data would suggest that a significant loss of body weight may be required before serum albumin concentration, and by inference net protein status, is impaired. In this population at least, changes in immune function measures were only apparent once serum albumin concentrations had dropped significantly below what may be considered a normal or healthy range.

It may be questioned whether the immune impairments observed in a number of these populations are justifiably attributed to protein-energy malnutrition alone. Nevertheless, appropriate nutritional intervention has been shown to alleviate many of the immune-suppressed functions in these individuals. Impaired cutaneous delayed hypersensitivity reactions were individually and collectively improved in malnourished children following nutritional treatment for 1–2 months.[20] The children were admitted to hospital and given up to 4 g protein/kg body weight/day, with the percentage of children with a positive response to a hypersensitivity test increasing from 14% on admission to 72% after 29 days of treatment. Elsewhere, it has been reported that specific lytic activity of natural killer cells increased from levels as low as 2.5% lysis to 12% lysis in children given nutritional support.[18] These data would affirm the contention that the impairments to cell-mediated immunity observed in these children were at least in part the direct result of malnutrition, and specifically protein deficiency.

4.2.2 Hospitalized Patients

A diet inadequate in protein content is not restricted to developing countries. Evidence for an important role of dietary protein for the functioning of the immune system has emerged from a number of studies of hospitalized patients in developed countries. The problem with drawing conclusions from patients who are both malnourished and seriously ill is the relative importance of nutritional and non-nutritional factors. Just as in the malnourished children, a number of studies have reported considerable improvement in immune-function indicators with nutritional support, even over reasonably short periods of time.[21] However, an evaluation of protein status, or serum albumin concentration, must be seen as essential if any meaningful comparison is to be made with an athletic population who might have only mild protein deficiencies.

In this regard, it is interesting to note that a number of authors refer to "clinically significant" malnutrition, and have attempted to develop guidelines of appropriate nutritional markers for its identification.[2,3] These have included serum albumin and transferrin as primary markers of nutritional status. Unfortunately, researchers have failed to agree on a value for serum albumin that is truly representative of a "clinically significant" nutritional status. Values as diverse as 21, 27, 28, 30, 32, 35 and 38 g/l have been cited in different studies.[3,21] Additionally, cutaneous delayed hypersensitivity tests have been widely used as an adjunct marker, based on the *a priori* assumption that poor nutritional status will impair this *in vivo* measure of immune status.[22] Prospective studies have found a combination of these three parameters to provide clinicians with a quantifiable index of malnutrition that will predict increased complications and mortality rates with some accuracy.[2]

One of the more comprehensive studies of immune-function parameters compared hospitalized patients with serum albumin levels below 32 g/l with a control group of hospitalized patients without nutritional deficiencies (serum albumin > 37 g/l).[21] Although there were no significant differences in serum immunoglobulin concentrations (IgG, IgM or IgA), it was once again the cell-mediated immunity that was negatively affected in the nutritionally deficient group. The response to cutaneous delayed hypersensitivity tests was significantly higher and T-lymphocyte proliferative responses to both pokeweed mitogen and PHA were between 4-fold and 10-fold higher, depending on the mitogen dose, in the nutritionally replete group. To underline the relative importance of protein malnutrition, protein repletion in the nutritionally deficient group produced a significant increase in T-lymphocyte response, restoring values to a similar magnitude to that observed in the control group. Unfortunately, the researchers did not report the serum albumin concentrations of the deficient group after refeeding to establish a required level of nutritional status for the restoration of T-lymphocyte function.[21]

4.2.3 The Elderly

Some of the most important data to relate immune-function status to protein nutritional status has emerged from studies of the elderly. Although the immune system has been reported to show an age-related response, it is equally true that nutritional deficiencies or undernourishment have been reported to occur in 30% of healthy aged subjects living at home.[23] In these populations, correlational analysis has suggested that immune responses and nutritional status of the elderly are inter-related, and significant evidence has been presented for a threshold for these effects.

Simultaneous assessments of nutritional parameters and immune function in the elderly have been reported.[24] A cohort of elderly men and women were separated into three groups on the basis of serum albumin concentrations (>35 g/l, 30–35 g/l, <30 g/l). Circulating concentrations of T-suppressor lymphocytes were unaffected by group, while significant decreases in circulating concentrations of T-helper lymphocytes were observed in both the 30–35 g/l and <30 g/l groups. All other immune parameters (total lymphocyte count, total T-lymphocyte count, lymphocyte proliferative response to PHA, and cutaneous delayed hypersensitivity tests) were significantly impaired in the <30 g/l group, but not in the 30–35 g/l group, when compared with the >35 g/l group.[24]

Other studies from the same group of researchers[25,26] have reported that elderly subjects (78.4 ± 9.3 years) with mild malnutrition (serum albumin 31.4 ± 3.7 g/l) had significantly lower T-lymphocyte and particularly T-helper lymphocyte circulating numbers, reduced lymphocyte proliferation responses, and cutaneous delayed hypersensitivity reactions than elderly (78.7 ± 7.4 years) subjects with normal serum albumin (42.1 ± 2.8 g/l) and healthy young adults (34.3 ± 13.7 years) with serum albumin concentrations of 43.3 ± 2.7 g/l. These data would suggest that the immune-function impairments observed during malnutrition, and particularly during an inadequate nutritional intake of protein, take effect at albumin concentrations below 30 g/l and possibly when levels are only between 30 and 35 g/l.[4]

4.2.4   Anorexia Nervosa

A final population that has been studied with regard to the effects of malnutrition on immune function has been those individuals with anorexia nervosa. They are unusual in that they are energy deficient, but with relatively few reports of increased incidences of infection. It has been suggested that anorexia nervosa is a consequence of a diet deficient in carbohydrate, yet adequate in protein and fat,[5,27] which may provide some protection from immune impairments in this population. Unfortunately, it is difficult to support this contention from the available literature, since most of the studies on the immune status of anorexic subjects do not provide information on the commonly recognized markers of nutritional status, such as serum albumin.

A notable exception has been a study reporting a group of anorexic subjects and a group of treated subjects who had regained weight over a 2-month period.[28] There were no significant differences in the immune variables measured. These included cutaneous delayed hypersensitivity tests, circulating numbers of T- and B-lymphocytes, serum concentrations of complement and immunoglobulins A, G, and M, and lymphocyte proliferative responses to PHA, pokeweed mitogen and concanavalin A. Importantly, these researchers reported that there were no significant differences between the serum albumin concentrations of the anorexia group (43 ± 6 g/l) and the treated group (42 ± 3 g/l), and none of the subjects would be classified as deficient in protein nutrition on the basis of this indicator. The normal immune variables in this particular study group may be attributable to the fact that protein availability was not impaired despite the reduced weight and total energy intake of the anorexia group. The paradox of anorexia, i.e., unlike other malnutrition conditions, increased incidences of infection are uncommon, may be attributable to sufficient protein availability, despite reduced total calorie intake.

Other authors have highlighted significant reductions in delayed hypersensitivity tests,[5,29] circulating numbers of lymphocytes,[29] T lymphocytes,[5,29] natural-killer cells, but not B-cells[29] of anorexic subjects when compared with healthy controls or those recovered from anorexia nervosa. Unfortunately, these authors did not report serum protein or serum albumin concentrations to enable a comparison of nutritional status. An important point raised by one of the authors[5] was that although no significant differences were observed in the peak lymphocyte responsiveness to mitogen, dose-response curves were shifted to the right in anorexic subjects. This indicated that a greater dose of mitogen was required to elicit a similar magnitude of T-lymphocyte response. It is an important methodological observation that this group had to use a detailed dose-response curve to uncover an abnormality in cell-mediated immunity. This change would have been undetected if peak responses alone had been investigated. So many of the lymphocyte proliferation studies only report peak responses. These data should be a good case in point to reform current methodology and adopt more appropriate approaches, if the clinical applications of these data are to be interpreted correctly.

4.2.5 Summary

There is clearly an association between an inadequacy of nutritional protein intake and an impaired cell-mediated immunity. Many fields of nutritional research and clinical practice have adopted an assessment of immunocompetence as a logical approach to the evaluation of nutritional, and particularly protein, status.[2, 3, 30] Furthermore, many studies have reported a restoration of cell-mediated immunity during periods of protein replenishment, further highlighting the essential requirement for sufficient dietary protein to support immune function.

However, it is equally clear that protein-energy malnutrition is not a discrete entity and should be seen to represent a spectrum of protein-deficient states, with the children of developing countries at one extreme and perhaps athletic populations at the other. The use of hypoalbuminemia as an indicator of malnutrition has been widely reported and may provide a useful link between the populations in which the immunosuppressive effects have been studied and observed and the athletic populations to which we wish to make application. Certainly, the consensus from the reported studies is that the effects of protein-deficient nutrition may not be apparent in immunosuppressive terms until serum albumin concentrations at least below 37 g/l have been reached. A word of caution has been reported:[3] Albumin may be quite stable in the face of short-term changes in nutritional status, and may require longer-term malnourishment to bring about a decrease in serum albumin concentrations. It has been suggested that thyroxin-binding pre-albumin and retinol-binding protein may give a better indication of rapid changes in nutritional status than albumin and transferrin, which may reflect longer-term malnutrition.[3] It may, therefore, be the case that longer-term deficiencies in protein intake are required to affect immune function, and cell-mediated immunity in particular, as they appear to be closely related to albumin concentration.

Indeed, a case could be made that the immunosuppressive effects of malnutrition are strongly related to the extent of albumin decrease in the elderly, in children from developing countries, in hospitalized patients, and in those with anorexia nervosa. There is also limited evidence that the immunosuppressive changes observed have clinical significance in that undernourished elderly with low serum albumin concentrations are far more likely to develop pulmonary infections than their well-nourished counterparts.[31] On this basis, it could be argued that immunosuppressive effects in athletes, mediated by a deficient nutritional protein intake, would only be apparent if similarly low serum albumin concentrations are observed during either acute exercise or chronic intensive and/or extensive training programs.

4.3   PROTEIN AND EXERCISE

It has been widely reported that athletes have an increased requirement for dietary protein intake, as a consequence of the exercise-induced increased rate of protein turnover.[32] Before attempting to evaluate any potential effects of nutritional protein deficit on immune function in athletes, a consideration of the level of protein requirement by athletes is essential. The evidence suggests that this requirement may differ depending on the nature of the training being undertaken.

4.3.1   Endurance Training

The increased requirement for dietary protein during endurance training is likely to be both as an auxiliary fuel source and to restore damaged muscle and other tissues. Evidence for an increased turnover of protein has been provided by both acute and chronic exercise studies. Some studies have simply reported an increased requirement for dietary protein during endurance exercise and training, while others have provided insight into whether athletes in general are meeting these requirements.

4.3.1.1   Acute Exercise

Evidence for an increased turnover of protein during acute exercise is provided by a number of studies that have reported an increased rate of protein, and particularly albumin, excretion in the urine post exercise. Reported increases in proteinuria are as high as 8- to 11-fold resting levels after competitive cycling or rowing exercise to exhaustion[33] and an increase in albuminuria of 20- to 25-fold after the same exercise. Overnight urinary excretion rates of albumin (4.6 ± 2.7 mg/min) have been reported to be similar between professional cyclists and non-athletes[34] but significantly increased following exercise (4.2 ± 2.6 vs. 18.1 ± 10.6 mg/min). The authors concluded that the recurrent excretion of protein, and in particularly albumin in the urine during exercise, may require an enhanced protein intake in athletes.

Even in moderate levels of physical activity, increased protein excretion has been reported. Lemon et al.[35] investigated the post-exercise urine urea nitrogen excretion following 1 h of exercise at approximately 40%, 55%, and 65% of $\dot{V}O_{2max}$ in healthy men. Significant elevations in nitrogen excretion were observed following the moderate and high-intensity exercise, but not following the low-intensity exercise, compared with a resting condition. Based on these data, they estimated that 1 h of moderate exercise increased protein oxidation by 29–45 g, therefore increasing nutritional requirements for protein by a similar amount. In glycogen-depleted states, the rate of protein oxidation during exercise may be more than twice that reported during a carbohydrate-loaded condition.[36]

Despite this increased turnover of protein during exercise, few studies have reported any significant decreases in biochemical markers of protein status. Concentrations of serum proteins immediately before and for 3 days after an ironman distance triathlon have been reported.[37] An initial concentration of 73.2 ± 3.4 g/l of serum protein did not change significantly either immediately after the 10-h race (75.8 ± 2.0 g/l) or during the following 3 days, with the lowest value being 68.5 ± 1.5 two days after the race. Immediately following a 42-km marathon run, significant increases in serum albumin have in fact been observed in 90 male and female competitors.[38] However, increases in serum albumin concentration following a bout of high-intensity exercise have been fully accounted for if corrected for exercise-induced plasma volume shifts,[39] issuing a caution to the interpretation of blood biochemistry immediately following acute exercise. These data would suggest that acute exercise, even of a prolonged duration, does not have a significant effect on serum indicators of protein status. Despite the increased requirement for protein during exercise, there is no evidence that this is sufficient in magnitude to have any effect on protein availability to the immune system. It may not be until recurrent bouts of exercise are undertaken and the cumulative effects of increased protein turnover are felt, that protein deficiency may be sufficient to impair immune function, if at all.[34]

4.3.1.2 Chronic Exercise

To gain an understanding of the protein requirements of endurance training, research studies have reported net nitrogen losses or gains when athletes were fed a known protein content in their diet. For example, a group of well-trained endurance runners, completing 12–16 km of running each day, were studied for a 6-day period.[40] When these athletes were fed a diet of 0.86 ± 0.23 g protein/kg body weight/day, they were estimated to be in negative nitrogen balance using urinary and sweat urea nitrogen loss. A second group of runners fed a diet with a higher protein content (1.49 ± 0.29 g/kg/day) were estimated to have a positive nitrogen balance (Figure 4.1A)

A separate study reported that 12 endurance runners of mixed age ranges were all in negative nitrogen balance over a 10-day period when fed a diet containing 0.6 g protein/kg body weight/day.[41] The authors estimated a protein requirement of 0.94

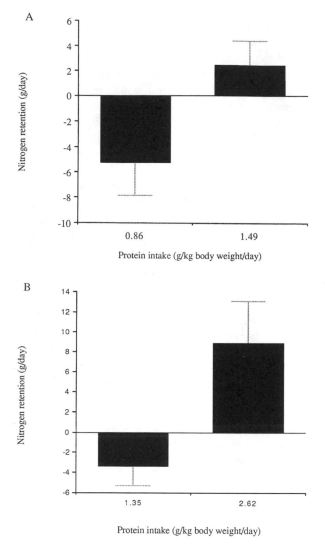

Figure 4. 1 Effect of dietary protein intake on nitrogen retention during endurance training (A) and resistance training (B). (Data from references 40, 48.)

± 0.05 g protein/kg body weight/day, while others have estimated that endurance athletes may require as much as 1.2–1.6 g protein/kg body weight/day,[32] which is approximately 1.5–2.0 times the recommended daily amount of 0.8 g protein/kg body weight/day. Given this increased level of dietary protein requirement, there is sufficient potential for athletes to become protein deficient following chronic training programs of extensive and/or intensive exercise. This may be a particular problem if a condition of glycogen depletion coexists with the training program, increasing protein oxidation as an auxiliary fuel.[36]

Conversely, the available evidence suggests that endurance athletes may very well be able to meet these requirements with some ease, since adequate protein intake has been reported in the diets of a number of athlete groups. Garcia-Roves et al.[42] reported on energy and protein intake during a 3-week professional cycling race, using weighed food records. They reported that the 10 cyclists were consuming 23.5 ± 1.8 MJ/day, which included more than 200 g protein per day, or 2.5–3.0 g/kg body weight/day. Evaluation of the dietary status of highly trained female cyclists, despite observing a moderate energy and carbohydrate deficiency, reported normal serum albumin levels (45 g/l) indicating that protein status was healthy.[43] One early study by Russian researchers has even suggested that serum concentrations of albumin and protein may increase during a period of training.[44]

4.3.1.3 *Overtraining*

A number of studies have assessed the effects of experimentally induced over-reaching or overtraining on serum indicators of protein status. In these studies, training volume has often been doubled over a 2- to 4-week period, which would clearly have a significant effect on the protein requirements of the body. However, only modest decreases in serum protein and albumin concentrations have been observed, if at all.[45-47] Gastmann et al.[45] reported serum albumin concentrations during a six-week period of intensive cycle ergometer training in six recreational athletes. Despite the training resulting in either stagnated or reduced performance in the athletes, no significant changes were observed in serum albumin, protein (69.4 vs. 68.7 g/l) or transferrin concentrations.

A study of elite soldiers involving 10 days of intensive training followed by six days of recovery produced considerable decreases in the performance of these athletes.[46] The authors reported that lymphocyte proliferative responses to con-canavalin A were decreased, although not significantly, following intensive training, and had decreased further during the recovery period. Despite this apparent decrease in immune status during training, serum concentrations of albumin were unaffected with the minimum concentration reported as 46.0 ± 0.8 g/l at the end of the 10-day training period (Figure 4.2). These data suggest that while intensive exercise programs may lead to a degree of immunosuppression, it is unlikely that this is a direct consequence of deficient nutritional supply of protein. Lehmann et al.[47] reported a longer 28-day period of increase training volume. During this time, total plasma protein concentrations only decreased from 78 ± 4.5 g/l before training to 72 ± 0.9 g/l at the end of the intensified training period. Serum albumin decreased significantly from 45.8 ± 1.3 g/l to 39.1 ± 3.1 g/l across the same time period. Even though these data suggest that if training is of a sufficient volume, biochemical markers of protein status can be observed to decrease, the absolute values still do not approach those previously associated with impaired immunocompetence.

4.3.2 RESISTANCE TRAINING

In some contrast to endurance training, resistance training is more likely to require an increased protein intake to provide amino acid availability as building

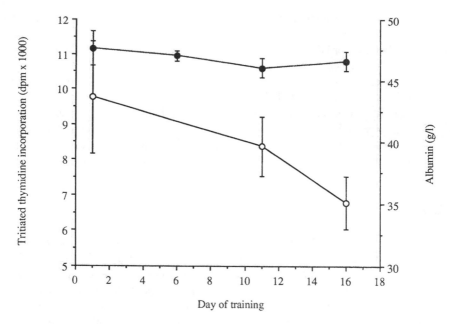

Figure 4.2 Effect of 10 days' overload training (days 1–10) and 6 days of recovery (days 11–16) on lymphocyte proliferation response (black dots) to the mitogen concanavalin A (as measured by tritiated thymidine incorporation) and serum albumin concentration (white dots). (Data from Reference 46.)

blocks for muscular development. Lemon et al.[48] repeated their earlier study of endurance runners using a group of men in the early stages of an intensive body-building training program. These athletes completed 1.5 hours of training 6 days/week for a one month period. One group consumed a diet containing 1.35 g protein/kg body weight/day and even with this level of protein intake were still estimated to be in negative nitrogen balance. A second group with a protein intake of 2.62 g protein/kg/day were estimated to be in positive nitrogen balance (Figure 4.1B).

These data lead the authors to make the recommendation that as much as 1.6–1.7 g protein/kg body weight/day may be required for athletes undergoing strength training programs.[48, 32] This estimate is more than twofold the WHO recommended daily protein requirement, and would clearly require a conscious effort on behalf of the athletes to maintain this level of nutritional intake. However, it is common practice among a large proportion of those athletes who undertake resistance training to supplement their diets with amino acid supplements. It has been reported that some athletes believe they require as much as 4.0–6.2 g protein/kg body weight/day during training.[32] Since these levels of nutritional intake are well in excess of those documented to be required,[48] it seems unlikely that protein deficiencies are a widespread problem in athletes undertaking resistance training.

4.4 CONCLUSIONS AND RECOMMENDATIONS

4.4.1 Effects of Exercise on Protein and Immunity

It is not surprising that protein deficiency is so consistently observed to interfere with resistance to infection because most immune mechanisms are dependent on cell replication or the production of active protein compounds. The real question though, which is still partially unanswered, is at what stage a protein deficiency is sufficient to have a demonstrable effect on immune function. There is no doubt that deterioration in immunity occurs in cases of severe protein deficiency, but is there a threshold below which effects are observed, or is it a case of a sliding scale of deficit?

Reconciling data collected in different population groups with so many confounding variables is inevitably problematic. Nevertheless, the available literature suggests that the effects of protein deficiency are not apparent from an immunological perspective until decreases in serum albumin concentration occur. Even the most conservative estimates have identified threshold values of serum albumin around 37–39 g/l, although many would argue that "clinically significant" effects of malnutrition are not felt until values as low as 30 g/l are reached. Concerns about protein-mediated immunodeficiencies in athletes would appear to be, in the main part at least, ill-founded. Neither during prolonged acute exercise, normal training regimes, or overload training and overtraining have serum albumin concentrations reached these established threshold levels, with perhaps one exception where levels of 39 g/l were reported.[47] Further studies may be required to establish any link between these mild changes in protein status and impaired immunity, since this has not been the specific area of interest in most studies where more-profound protein deficiencies are more common.

4.4.2 Effects of Infection on Protein and Exercise

The opposite side of the protein, exercise, and immunity argument also warrants some discussion. Infections, particularly those of a severe nature or of a long duration, have been observed to be associated with profound changes in protein metabolism and turnover. Serum albumin concentrations, for example, are known to be decreased in a variety of different types of infection,[49] with greater decreases observed during more-severe infectious episodes. This decrease is probably a reflection of a reduced rate of protein synthesis, an increased rate of degradation or a combination of the two processes. Since albumin is thought to serve as a storage form of amino acid, changes in serum albumin concentration may reflect a process of making amino acids available for the synthesis of other critically needed protein for immune function.

The average protein loss during infection is of the order of 0.6 g protein/kg body weight/day. This is almost equal to the mean estimated protein requirement for sedentary adults. During more-severe infections, such as typhoid fever, protein losses have been reported to reach as high as 1.2 g protein/kg body weight/day.[49] For an athlete who may be immunosuppressed by whatever means, an infection has the potential to initiate a vicious cycle of interrelated events: An impaired immune system, whether through protein insufficiency or not, may provide an opening for opportunistic infections. In turn, infections will result in an increased utilization of protein, reduced serum protein and albumin concentrations, and a reduction in the availability of protein, which could further compromise the immune system. Infected athletes who attempt to maintain any form of training program may place themselves into an increasingly immunocompromised state, as the immune system and the exercising muscles represent competing demands for the decreasingly available protein.

4.4.3 Nutritional Recommendations

The majority of studies have reported that while protein requirements of athletes are elevated above the WHO recommendation of 0.8 g protein/kg body weight/day, most athletes are able to meet this requirement with some ease. The consensus has been that endurance athletes may require between 1.2–1.6 g protein/kg body weight/day,[32] while athletes undertaking resistance training may need to increase this to 1.6–1.7 g protein/kg body weight/day.[48] Because these levels of protein intake should be sufficient to maintain protein balance, they should be adequate to prevent any protein-mediated immunosuppressive effects. Perhaps the one area of concern would be in those athletes who are glycogen depleted as a result of recurrent bouts of intensive and/or extensive training, as protein oxidation is known to increase during exercise in the absence of available carbohydrate.[36] There has been a great deal of interest in the possibility that supplementing the diet of athletes with specific amino acids will improve immune function and provide a resistance to infection. While a good deal of work has shown beneficial effects in those individuals with protein-energy malnutrition, little work has been able to prove an additional effect in those individuals with a healthy nutritional status.[14]

REFERENCES

1. Chandra, R.K., Nutrition and the immune system: an introduction, *Am. J. Clinical Nutr.*, 66, 460S, 1997.
2. Buzby, G.P., Mullen, J.L., Matthews, D.C., Hobbs, C.L. and Rosato, E.F., Prognostic nutritional index in gastrointestinal surgery, *Am. J. Surg.*, 139, 160, 1980.
3. Linn, B.S., A protein-energy malnutrition scale (PEMS), *Ann. Surg.*, 200, 747, 1984.
4. Lesourd, B., Protein undernutrition as the major cause of decreased immune function in the elderly: clinical and functional implications, *Nutr. Rev.*, 53, S86, 1995.
5. Cason, J., Ainley, C.C., Wolstencrofy, R.A., Norton, K.R. and Thompson, R.P., Cell-mediated immunity in anorexia nervosa, *Clinical and Experimental Immun.* 64, 370, 1986.
6. Lemon, P.W., Effect of exercise on dietary protein requirements, *Int. J. Sport Nutr.*, 8, 426, 1998.
7. Nieman, D.C., Johanssen, L.M., Lee, J.W. and Arabatzis, K., Infectious episodes in runners before and after the Los Angeles marathon, *J. Sports Med.*, 30, 316, 1990.
8. Peters, E.M. and Bateman, E.D., Ultramarathon running and upper respiratory tract infection. *S. Afr. Med. J.*, 64, 582, 1983.

9. Heath, G.W., Ford, E.S., Craven, T.E., Macrea, C.A., Jackson, K.L. and Pate, R.E., Exercise and the incidence of upper respiratory tract infection, *Med. and Scien. in Sports and Exerc.*, 23, 152, 1991.

10. Hodges, R.E., Bean, W.B., Ohlson, M.A. and Bleiler, R.E., Factors affecting human antibody response I: Effects of variations in dietary protein upon the antigenic response of men, *Am. J. Clinical Nutr.*, 10, 500, 1962.

11. Chandra, R.K., Lymphocyte subpopulations in human malnutrition: cytotoxic and suppressor cells, *Pediatrics*, 59, 423, 1977.

12. Rikimaru, T., Taniguchi, K., Yartey, J.E., Kennedy, D.O., and Nkrumah, F.K., Humoral and cell-mediated immunity in malnourished children in Ghana, *Eur. J. Clinical Nutr.*, 52, 344, 1998.

13. Schopfer, K. and Douglas, S.D., *In vitro* studies of lymphocytes from children with kwashiorkor. *Clinical Immun.*, 5, 21, 1976.

14. Scrimshaw, N.S. and SanGiovanni, J.P., Synergism of nutrition, infection, and immunity: an overview, *Am. J. Clinical Nutr.*, 66, 464S, 1997.

15. Martin, T.R., The relationship between malnutrition and lung infections, *Clinics in Chest Med.*, 8, 359, 1987.

16. Kirsch, R., Frith, L., Black, E., and Hoffenberg, R., Regulation of albumin synthesis and catabolism by alteration of dietary protein, *Nature*, 217, 578, 1968.

17. Salimonu, L.S., Ojo-Amaize, E., Williams, A., Johnson, A., Cooke, A., Adekunle, F., Alm, G., and Wigzell, H., Depressed natural killer cell activity in children with protein-calorie malnutrition, *Clinical Immun. and Immunopathology*, 24, 1, 1982.

18. Salimonu, L.S., Ojo-Amaize, E., Johnson, A., Laditan, A., Akinwolere, O., and Wigzell, H., Depressed natural killer cell activity in children with protein-calorie malnutrition, *Cellular Immun.*, 82, 210, 1983.

19. Nieman, D.C., Buckley, K.S., Henson, D.A., Warren, B.J., Suttles, J., Ahle, J.C., Simandle, S., Fagoaga, O.R., and Nehlsen-Cannarella, S.L., Immune function in marathon runners vs. sedentary controls, *Med. and Sci. in Sports and Exerc.*, 27, 986, 1995.

20. Edelman, R., Suskind, R., Olson, R.E., and Sirisinha, S., Mechanisms of defensive delayed cutaneous hypersensitivity in children with protein-calorie malnutrition, *Lancet*, 1, 506, 1973.

21. Law, D.K., Dudrick, S.J., and Arbou, N.I., Immunocompetence of patients with protein-calorie malnutrition, *Ann. of Intern. Med.*, 79, 545, 1973.

22. Mullen, J.L., Gertner, M.H., Buzby, G.P., Goodhart, G.L., and Rosato, E.F., Implications of malnutrition in the surgical patient, *Arch. Surg.*, 114, 121, 1979.

23. Dirren, H., Decarli, B., Lesourd, B., Schlienger, J.L., Deslypere, J.P., and Kiepurski, A., Nutritional status: haematology and albumin, *Eur. J. Clinical Nutr.*, 45, 43, 1991.

24. Lesourd, B., Moulias, R., Favre-berrone, M., and Rapin, C.H., Nutritional influences on immune responses in the elderly, in *Nutr. and Immun.*, Chandra, C.K., Eds., ARTS Biomedical Publishers, St. Johns, Nfld. (Canada), 1992, 211.

25. Lesourd, B., La dénutrition protéique: principale cause de deficit immunitaire chez sujet age, *Age Nutr.*, 1, 132, 1990.

26. Lesourd, B.M, Nutrition and immunity in the elderly: modification of immune responses with nutritional treatments, *Am. J. Clinical Nutr.*, 66, 478S, 1997.

27. Russell, G.F.M., The nutritional disorder in anorexia nervosa, *J. Psychosomatic Res.*, 11, 141, 1967.

28. Golla, J.A., Larson, L.A., Anderson, C.F., Lucas, A.R., Wilson, W.R., and Tomasi, T.B., An immunological assessment of patients with anorexia nervosa, *Am. J. Clinical Nutr.*, 34, 2756, 1981.

29. Marcos, A., Varela, P., Toro, O., Lopez-Vidriero, I., Nova, E., Madruga, D., Casas, J., and Morande, G., Interactions between nutrition and immunity in anorexia nervosa: a 1-y follow-up study, *Am. J. Nutr.*, 66, 485S, 1997.

30. Chandra, R.K., Immunocompetence as a functional index for nutritional status, *Brit. Med. Bull.*, 37, 89, 1981.

31. Scrimshaw, N.S., Tatlor, C.E., and Gordon, J.E., Interactions of nutrition and infection, *Nutrition*, 4, 13, 1988.

32. Lemon, P.W.R., Effects of exercise on dietary protein requirements, *Int. J. Sports Nutr.*, 8, 426, 1998.

33. Poortmans, J.R., Jourdain, M., Heyters, C., and Reardon, F.D., Postexercise proteinuria in rowers, *Can. J. Sports Sci.*, 15, 126, 1990.

34. Clerico, A., Giammattei, C., Cecchini, L., Lucchetti, A., Cruschelli, L., Penno, G., Gregori, G., and Giampietro, O., Exercise-induced proteinuria in well-trained athletes, *Clinical Chem.*, 36, 562, 1990.

35. Lemon, P.W., Dolny, D.G., and Yarasheski, K.E., Moderate physical activity can increase dietary protein needs, *Can. J. App. Physiol.*, 22, 494, 1997.

36. Lemon, P.W. and Mullin, J.P., Effect of initial muscle glycogen levels on protein catabolism during exercise, *J. App. Physiol.*, 48, 624, 1980.

37. Fellmann, N., Sagnol, M., Bedu, M., Falgairette, G., Van Praagh, E., Gaillard, G., Jouanel, P., and Coudert, J., Enzymatic and hormonal responses following a 24 h endurance run and a 10 h triathlon race, *Eur. J. App. Physiol.*, 57, 545, 1988.

38. Weight, L.M., Alexander, D., and Jacobs, P., Strenuous exercise: analogous to the acute-phase response? *Clinical Sci.*, 81, 677, 1991.

39. Kargotich, S., Goodman, C., Keast, D., Fry, R.W., Garcia-Webb, P., Crawford, P.M., and Morton, A.R., Influence of exercise-induced plasma volume changes on the interpretation of biochemical data following high-intensity exercise, *Clinical J. Sports Med.*, 7, 185, 1997.

40. Friedman, J.E. and Lemon, P.W., Effect of chronic endurance exercise on retention of dietary protein, *Int. J. Sports Med.*, 10, 118, 1989.

41. Meredith, C.N., Zachin, M.J., Frontera, W.R., and Evans, W.J., Dietary protein requirements and body protein metabolism in endurance-trained men, *J. App. Physiol.*, 66, 2850, 1989.

42. Garcia-Roves, P.M., Terrados, N., Fernandez, S.F., and Patterson, A.M., Macronutrients intake of top level cyclists during continuous competition – change in the feeding pattern, *Int. J. Sports Med.*, 19, 61, 1998.

43. Keith, R.E., O'Keeffe, K.A., Alt, L.A., and Young, K.L., Dietary status of trained female cyclists, *J. Am. Dietetic Assoc.*, 89, 1620, 1989.

44. Efimenko, A.M., Tolkacheva, N.V., Ostolovskii, E.M., and Stanevich, A.V., Blood serum proteins during sports training, *Ukrainskii Biokhimicheskii Zhurnal*, 50, 723, 1978.

45. Gastmann, U., Petersen, K.G., Bocker, J., and Lehmann, M., Monitoring intensive endurance training at moderate energetic demands using resting laboratory markers failed to recognize an early overtraining stage, *J. Sports Med. and Physical Fitness*, 38, 188, 1998.

46. Fry, R.W., Morton, A.R., Garcia-Webb, P., Crawford, G.P.M., and Keast, D., Biological responses to overload training in endurance sports, *Eur. J. Appl. Physiol.*, 64, 335, 1992.

47. Lehmann, M., Dickhuth, H.H., Gendrisch, G., Lazar, W., Thum, M., Kaminski, R., Aramendi, J.F., Peterke, E., Wieland, W., and Keul, J., Training — overtraining; a prospective, experimental study with experienced middle- and long-distance runners, *Int. J. Sports Med.*, 12, 444, 1991.
48. Lemon, P.W., Tarnopolsky, M.A., MacDougall, J.D., and Atkinson, S.A., Protein requirements and muscle mass/strength changes during intensive training in novice bodybuilders, *J. Appl. Physiol.*, 73, 767, 1992.
49. Powanda, M.C., Changes in body balances of nitrogen and other key nutrients: description and underlying mechanisms, *Am. J. Clinical Nutr.*, 30, 1254, 1977.

CHAPTER 5

Glutamine, Exercise, and the Immune System

Thomas Rohde, Kenneth Ostrowski, and Bente Klarlund Pedersen

CONTENTS

5.1 INTRODUCTION

Although it has generally been accepted that cells of the immune system obtain their energy through the metabolism of glucose,[1] it has also been established that glutamine is an important energy source for lymphocytes and macrophages.[2] Several lines of evidence suggest that glutamine is used at a very high rate by these cells, even when they are quiescent,[3] and it has been proposed that the glutamine pathway in lymphocytes may be under external regulation, due partly to the supply of glutamine itself.[4] As skeletal muscle is the major tissue involved in glutamine production and known to release glutamine into the blood stream at a high rate, it has been suggested that skeletal muscle plays a vital role in maintenance of the rate of the key process of glutamine utilization by cells of the immune system. Consequently, the activity of the skeletal muscle may directly influence the immune system.

1-8493-0741-4/00/$0.00+$.50
© 2000 by CRC Press LLC

It has been hypothesized that during intense physical exercise, or in relation to surgery, trauma, burn, and sepsis, the demands on muscle and other organs for glutamine are so high that the immune system may suffer from a lack of glutamine that temporarily affects its function.[3,5,6] Thus, factors that directly or indirectly influence glutamine synthesis or release could theoretically influence the function of lymphocytes and monocytes.[3,5]

The glutamine hypothesis may have important clinical implications in relation to exercise immunology. Several studies have shown that strenuous exercise is followed by changes in concentrations and function of blood mononuclear cells as measured by *in vitro* and *in vivo* immunological methods. Thus, following prolonged intense exercise, the number of lymphocytes in the blood is depressed below pre-values, and the functions of natural-killer (NK) and B cells are impaired.[7] Further-more, exercise inhibits mucosal immunity.[8] Several epidemiological studies suggest that intense exercise of long duration is associated with increased risk of upper respiratory tract infection (URTI) symptoms.[9] Also, epidemiological and experimen-tal studies show that during the incubation period of an infection, depending on the pathogen, exercise may worsen the disease outcome.[10]

While significant changes in the concentration and functional activity of some immune parameters might be observed, they may not necessarily manifest into higher incidence of infections and illness. In other words, it has not formally been proven that immune changes in relation to acute exercise provide the physiological rationale for increased frequency of post-exercise URTI symptoms. However, when the immune system was evaluated by *in vivo* immunological methods, including eval-uation of the cell-mediated immune response by the delayed type hypersensitivity skin test response to certain recall antigens, the cumulative skin test responses were significantly lower in subjects performing strenuous exercise (a triathlon race) than in untrained and trained control groups. The finding that *in vivo* cell-mediated immunity was impaired in the first days after prolonged high-intensity exercise indicates that post-exercise immune impairment measured by *in vitro* methods could be of clinical significance.

In this review, the potential role of glutamine in the post-exercise (*in vitro*) immunosuppression and the value of glutamine as a nutritional supplement to ath-letes are discussed.

5.2 GLUTAMINE METABOLISM

Glutamine has been classified as a non-essential amino acid based on studies showing that it was not required as a dietary nutrient.[11] In 1955, when Harry Eagle found that glutamine was an essential nutrient for cells in culture, it was recognized that it might have important metabolic properties.[12,13]

Glutamine, the most abundant amino acid in the human body, is a neutral glycogenic amino acid. The normal plasma concentration is 500–700 mM and in human skeletal muscle the concentration is 20 mM.[14] Glutamine is available in the lumen of the intestine in the form of peptides derived from protein and can be taken up by the absorptive cells of the intestine. However, these cells utilize glutamine at

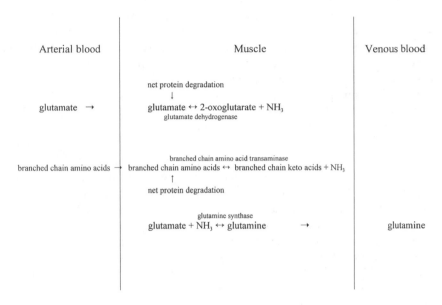

Figure 5.1 Glutamine synthesis in skeletal muscle.

a high rate and probably use up most of the absorbed glutamine, leaving only small amounts to enter the circulation.[15] To accomplish the high demands for glutamine in the body, it is synthesized by several organs, including skeletal muscles, kidneys, liver, lungs, and heart. Arterio-venous difference measurements indicate that skeletal muscle is the most important site for glutamine synthesis.[3,6] Skeletal muscle has high activities of branched chain amino acid (BCAA) transaminase and glutamine synthase, which are key enzymes in the synthesis of glutamine. Glutamine is produced from glutamate and ammonia catalyzed by glutamine synthase. In the muscle, glutamate can be obtained from protein degradation or from the combination of 2-oxoglutarate (a citric cycle intermediate) and BCAA (leucine, isoleucine and valine), catalyzed by BCAA transaminase. Furthermore, glutamate can be taken up from the circulation. The necessary ammonia can be obtained from the free pool of ammonia or donated from the BCAA's via deamination (Figure 5.1)

5.3 ROLES OF GLUTAMINE

As energy supply, glutamine has been shown to be important for tumor cells and enterocytes.[16] A high rate of glutamine utilization characterizes a number of different cells (tumor cells, fibroblasts, and cells of the immune system). Based on the activities of a number of key enzymes, it has been shown that lymphocytes and macrophages have a high capacity to use glutamine. Furthermore, the rate of glutamine utilization by these cells is either similar to or greater than that of glucose both when the cells are active and quiescent. While mononuclear cells have a high intracellular activity of glutaminase, they do not possess the ability to synthesize glutamine in that they have no activity of glutamine synthase. This has been shown by direct measurement of the enzyme [17] and by indirect measurement of the capability of lymphocytes to produce glutamine.[18] The consequence of this is that lymphocytes must be supplied with glutamine in the plasma to accomplish the metabolic requirements. As skeletal muscles contain the largest store of glutamine in the body, release of glutamine from skeletal muscles is thought to be the main source to maintain the plasma glutamine concentration.

Although there is high utilization of both glucose and glutamine, the oxidation of these compounds is only partial. The major end product of glucose metabolism is lactate, and of glutamine metabolism they are glutamate, lactate, and aspartate.[6] A high rate of glutamine utilization, but only partial oxidation characterizes several types of cells, described in tumor cells by McKeehan, who termed the process glutaminolysis.[19] The high rate of glutamine utilization, but only partial oxidation does not speak in favor of glutamine's proving to be a major supply of energy. If the role of glutaminolysis were solely to provide energy, it would be expected that the carbon skeleton would be completely oxidized by the citric acid cycle. Thus, a quantitative theory of metabolic control to branched pathways has been applied to explain the high rate of glutamine utilization by lymphocytes and macrophages. If the flux through one branch is largely in excess of the other, then the sensitivity of the flux in the low-flux pathway to specific regulators is very high. Hence, in rapidly dividing and proliferating cells, high rates of glutaminolysis (and glycolysis) are required not for energy or precursor provision per se but for high sensitivity of the biosynthetic pathways involved in the use of precursors for macromolecular synthesis (e.g., the synthesis of DNA and RNA). According to this theory, the high rate of utilization provides a sensitive but stable system that allows cells to multiply very fast in response to a challenge, e.g., the lymphocyte proliferative response in relation to a viral infection.

5.4 PLASMA GLUTAMINE CONCENTRATIONS AND ACUTE EXERCISE

The concentration of glutamine in plasma has been reported to decline in relation to trauma, sepsis, and burns.[20] Furthermore, several studies have shown that in relation to intense sustained exercise the plasma glutamine concentration decreases,[21-25] whereas few studies have shown no changes in plasma glutamine.[26,27] Skeletal muscles are the major sites for glutamine production[6] and an increase in the release of glutamine resulting in a decrease in the intracellular concentration has been shown to occur in relation to the above-mentioned stress situations. However, the decrease in plasma glutamine concentration, despite the increased release from skeletal muscle, is not well understood. The decrease in plasma glutamine concentration is without doubt due to net overutilization, which is probably the result either of increased amino acid extraction by the liver (for gluconeogenesis and urea formation),[28] or of an increased rate of glutamine utilization by the kidneys and cells of the immune system.[3] In relation to long-term exercise, and in overtrained athletes, another theory is that these conditions interfere with the rate of glutamine release from muscles and thus could be responsible for the decrease in the plasma glutamine concentration.[3]

The changes in glutamine concentrations vary depending on the type, duration, and intensity of exercise (see Table 5.1). However, the majority of studies concerning changes in glutamine in relation to exercise indicates that there is a transient decrease in the period following both acute exercise and in the overtraining syndrome. In relation to other forms of stress, decreases in the plasma glutamine concentration have been reported.[29,30] It is important to note that the largest decrease is reported after major burns (>30% of total body surface) with the plasma glutamine concentration declining from 490 mM to 200 mM.[30]

5.5 PLASMA GLUTAMINE CONCENTRATIONS AND OVERTRAINING

Recently, it was shown that resting plasma glutamine concentrations in athletes vary between sports. That is, plasma glutamine concentrations were higher in cyclists, but lower in powerlifters and swimmers.[31] The latter finding may be ascribed to different metabolic demands of the different sports. Low chronic plasma glutamine concentrations have been described in relation to overtraining.[32–34] Another study on swimmers found that plasma glutamine levels did not decrease during periods of intensified training, and that appearance of URTIs were not related to changes in plasma glutamine concentrations in overtrained swimmers.[35]

5.6 GLUTAMINE AND *IN VITRO* IMMUNE FUNCTION

The initial finding of Eagle[12,13] that glutamine is an essential nutrient for cells replicating in culture has been extended to many different cell types. It is recognized that glutamine is an important tissue culture supplement, necessary for the survival and growth of a variety of mammalian cells[19,20,36,37] including cells of the immune system.[2,38] Furthermore, it has been shown that other amino acids, combinations of glutamate and ammonia or combinations of glutamate and leucine cannot substitute for glutamine.[17, 18] Glutamine influences the *in vitro* proliferation of human lymphocytes when stimulated with ConA,[18,30,39] PHA,[18,39] IL-2,[18,39] or purified protein derivative of Mycobacterium Tuberculosis (PPD)[39] in a concentration-dependent manner with optimal proliferation at a glutamine concentration around the physiological level (600 mM). Even at lower glutamine concentrations (between 100 and 300 mM) the proliferation is still augmented. The influence of glutamine on the proliferative response of lymphocytes has also been examined in rats,[2] and similar results have been obtained with optimal proliferation at glutamine concentrations of approximately 300 mM.[2] Wallace and Keast[40] used a thymocyte assay to show that the secretion of IL-1 by murine macrophages in response to LPS stimulation was dependent on the availability of glutamine in the culture medium. Calder and Newsholme[41] showed that the presence of glutamine in the medium of ConA-stimulated rat lymphocytes enhanced the production of IL-2 (measured by bioassay).

Table 5.1 Changes in Glutamine Concentrations in Relation to Various Forms of Exercise

Author	Exercise type	n	Sample type	Gln. conc. μM	Gln. conc. μM	P<
Parry-Billings 1992	overtrained	40	ven. plasma	controls: 550	subjects: 503	0.02
	marathon	24	ven. plasma	pre:592	immed. post: 495	0.001
	marathon (+BCAA)	23	ven. plasma	pre: 581	immed. post: 561	NS
	30-km treadmill run	12	ven. plasma	pre: 641	immed. post: 694	NS
	cycling (73% VO_{2max})	4	ven. plasma	pre: 641	immed. post: 615	NS
	sprints (10x6s)	10	ven. plasma	pre: 556	immed. post: 616	0.05
Lehmann 1995	ultra-triathlon	9	serum	pre: 500	immed. post: 497	NS
Castell 1997	marathon	12	ven. plasma	pre: 571	immed. post: 462	0.001
Rohde 1996	triathlon	8	serum	pre: 468	post: 2h: 318	0.05
Rohde 1997	repeated exer. 60, 45, 30 min at 75% VO_{2max}, separated by 2 h rest	8	art. plasma	pre: 508	post 2h (last exer. bout): 402	0.05
Rohde 1997	marathon	8	ven. plasma	pre: 647	post 1.5 h: 470	0.0001
Keast 1995	15x1 min treadmill run (120% VO_{2max}) Overtraining	5	ven.plasma	pre: 630	day 11: 328	0.08

We found[18] that IL-2 and IFN-g production by PHA-stimulated human blood mononuclear cells, measured by ELISA kits, were enhanced by the presence of glutamine at a concentration of 600 mM, whereas the production of IL-1β, IL-6 or TNF-α was not influenced by glutamine (see Table 5.2). Thus, it is possible that glutamine could influence lymphocyte proliferation by inducing the production of IL-2 and IFN-γ.

The *in vitro* influence of glutamine on the cytotoxic activity of human lymphocytes was investigated in a study from our laboratory.[39] When blood mononuclear cells were incubated for 48 hours in the presence of IL-2, with or without glutamine, and tested for LAK cell activity in a ^{51}Cr-release assay, it was shown that the presence of glutamine augmented the LAK activity with optimal lysis at a glutamine concentration of 300 mM. The increase in LAK activity was apparently not due to more LAK cells in the assay, as glutamine did not influence the percentage of CD16+ and CD56+ cells in an experiment where BMNC were stimulated with IL-2. In contrast

Table 5.2   IL-2, IFN-γ, IL-1β, IL–6, and TNF–α Measured by ELISA in Supernatants from LPS- and PHA-Stimulated BMNC

	gln 1	gln 2	glu	glu/leu	control
IL-2 (24h)	1038±173***	1056±160***	225±84	236±60	247±30
IFN-γ (24h)	1940±361**	2035±455**	1304±423	968±252	1182±31
IFN-γ (48h)	2840±511	2708±483*	1707±452	1390±403	1643±441
IL-1β (4h)	7823±1117	8115±1220	6872±859	7344±1028	6804±974
IL-1β (24h)	20527±2023	17454±2591	19793±2449	19381±2423	18800±2099
IL–6 (4h)	1983±210	1852±179	1961±208	1890±184	1931±179
IL–6 (24h)	8085±947	7778±997	8257±824	8772±1154	7577±699
TNF–α (24h)	2228±557	2082±503	2026±463	2104±514	2218±690
TNF–α (24h)	2314±563	2160±619	1662±374	1824±505	1829±440

to the relationship between LAK cell activity and glutamine concentration, the function of NK cells was not influenced by glutamine. The supportive role of glutamine in the generation of LAK-cell activity has also been found by Juretic et al.,[42] who discovered that glutamine deficit affected the LAK cell activity by limiting the number of generated effector cells while acquisition of broad-range killing was not affected. Fahr et al[43] also found a relationship between glutamine and IL-2-primed LAK cells. Furthermore, in relation to a triathlon, the time course of changes in serum glutamine concentration were paralleled by changes in LAK-cell activities (positive correlation between LAK-cell activity and serum glutamine concentration, r=0.39, $P<0.01$).[24]

5.7 GLUTAMINE SUPPLEMENTATION, EXERCISE, AND IMMUNE FUNCTION

Several studies have examined the effect of glutamine as a part of total parenteral nutrition (TPN), on cells of the immune system and on the function of the intestine in both humans and rats. In humans, it has been shown that glutamine-enriched intravenous feeding to patients with haematological malignancies in remission (after high-dose chemotherapy and total body irradiation) decreased the amount of positive microbial culture and diminished the number of clinical infections.[44] Studies in rats have shown that addition of glutamine to TPN abolished the suppressed level of biliary IgA observed in relation to standard TPN, and thus may offer protection against bacterial translocation from the gut.[45] Yoshida et al.[46] showed that, when glutamine was added to standard TPN, the rate of hepatic regeneration following partial hepatectomy in rats was increased due to increased protein synthesis in the liver and increased DNA synthesis in hepatocytes. In septic rats, it was shown that glutamine-supplemented TPN diminished the increase of urea production, partially prevented the decrease in lymphocyte blastogenesis, and increased the phagocytic index as compared with standard TPN.[47] Fahr et al.[43] showed that oral glutamine supplementation of tumor-bearing rats decreased the tumor growth, which was associated with an increase in IL-2-primed LAK-cell activity. These studies were based on the fact that, in rats, TPN induces intestinal villus atrophy and an increased permeability of the intestine. However, in humans, Buchmann et al.[48] found that the changes in the intestine resulting from TPN were substantially less significant than the changes occurring in rats, and in another study[49] they found that TPN was not associated with intestinal immune dysfunction. A recent study by Shewchuck[50] evaluated the influence of regular exercise and dietary glutamine supplementation in rats and found no effect of glutamine supplementation on immune function. Koyama et al.[51] showed that chronic exercise in rats resulted in decreased plasma glutamine concentrations paralleled by decreased concanavalin-A stimulated T-lymphocyte proliferation. The same relationship was shown when glutamine synthesis was inhibited by injection of methionine sulfoximine, indicating an association between glutamine and T-cell proliferation.

Using a triathlon model, it was found that the decline in plasma glutamine was correlated to the decline in LAK cell activity.[24] In another study using an 8-week aerobic or anaerobic training model, a correlation was found between the decrease in plasma glutamine and the decline in number of CD4+ cells. However, this relationship was shown only in the anaerobic training group.[52]

Few studies have been performed to investigate whether supplementation of glutamine to endurance athletes to abolish post-exercise decline in plasma glutamine concentration has an effect on post-exercise immunosuppression. Castell et al.[53] supplemented runners participating in ultramarathons, marathons, 10-km races, or 15-mile training sessions and rowers undertaking circuit training for 1 h or 5 km ergometer rowing. The athletes received 5 g L-glutamine or placebo on a double-blind basis. The glutamine supplementation was given in two doses, one immediately after exercise and a second dose 2 h later. The decrease in plasma glutamine in the placebo group after exercise was reported to be between 12% and 20%. Based on questionnaires, 80.8% of the glutamine-supplemented marathon runners reported no infections in the 7 days post-exercise, compared with 48.8 % in the placebo group. In contrast, Mackinnon et al.[35] showed no significant difference in glutamine levels between subjects who did or did not develop URTI in a study examining the effect of intensified training on swimmers. Furthermore, it was shown that the plasma glutamine concentration did not necessarily decrease during periods of intensified training.

Another placebo-controlled study by Castell et al.[54] showed that glutamine supplementation to runners after a marathon race did not influence the lymphocyte distribution or the plasma concentration of IL-6, IFN-γ or CRP. In the latter study, glutamine was supplemented immediately after and 1 h after the end of exercise. However, in order to prevent a decrease in the plasma glutamine concentration, glutamine has to be supplemented approximately every 30 min[25] and it is dubious whether the glutamine supplementation in the above-mentioned studies was sufficient to avoid a decrease in the plasma glutamine concentration. This is emphasized by the fact that the plasma glutamine concentration in both the glutamine-supplemented and the placebo group in the latter study actually declined significantly (to a similar level).

glutamine concentration

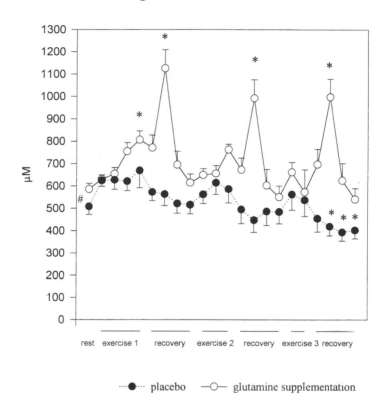

Figure 5.2 Arterial plasma glutamine concentration in the placebo and the glutamine supplementation trial. *Notes:* *Significant difference from resting value in each trial, p<0.05. #Significant difference between trials, p<0.05. (From Reference 25)

Well-trained athletes performing repeated bicycle-ergometer exercise in a blind crossover, randomized, placebo-controlled study were supplemented with glutamine.[25] The athletes performed 60, 45, and 30 min exercise at 75% of maximal oxygen consumption separated by 2 h resting periods. Glutamine (100 mg per kg body weight) was supplemented 30 min prior to the end, at the end, and 30 min after each exercise bout. Arterial plasma glutamine concentration declined from 508±35 (pre-exercise) to 402±38 mM (2 h after the last exercise bout) in the placebo trial. Glutamine was maintained above pre-exercise level at all time points in the glutamine supplementation trial (see Figure 5.2). There were no differences between the two trials in the concentration of lymphocytes, leukocyte subpopulations, lymphocyte proliferation, LAK activity or NK activity. Thus, glutamine supplementation did not abolish the post-exercise immunosuppression characterized by a decrease in lymphocyte concentration and a decrease in the LAK-cell activity. Comparable results were found in a field study (randomized, placebo controlled)[23] showing that glutamine supplementation to marathon runners did not influence the exercise-induced immunological changes. Venous

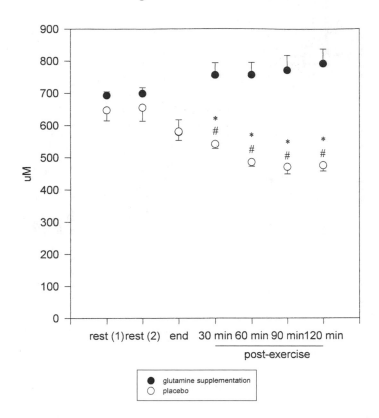

Figure 5.3   Plasma glutamine concentration in the glutamine-supplemented and the placebo
group. *Note*: #Significant difference between the glutamine-supplemented and the
placebo group, p<0.05. *Significant difference from rest, p<0.05. Rest (1): blood
samples taken one week prior to the race; rest (2): blood samples taken the day
before the race. (From Reference 23)

plasma glutamine concentration declined from 647mM pre-race to 470 mM, 120 min
post-race in the placebo group whereas plasma glutamine concentration was maintained
in the glutamine supplementation group (see Figure 5.3). In this study, no difference in
lymphocyte proliferation was observed between the glutamine and the placebo group,
whereas glutamine addition *in vitro* enhanced the proliferative response equally in the
two groups. This demonstrates and confirms that glutamine as a culture supplement is
capable of enhancing the proliferation response but indicates that the influence of
glutamine *in vitro* is not dependent on the plasma concentration of glutamine.

In a recent double-blind placebo-controlled study, glutamine supplementation
was performed during and after 2 h concentric bicycle exercise at 75% of VO_{2max}.
Decreased lymphocyte concentration, decreased proliferative response, and decrease
in NK- and LAK-cell activity were found. Furthermore, decreased concentration of
IgA in saliva (total and relative to total protein) as well as decreased IgA output was

found in response to exercise. Also, following bicycle exercise, there was an increase in IL-6. However, glutamine supplementation did not influence any of these parameters (Pedersen, B.K., unpublished results).

5.8 DISCUSSION

The hypothesis stating that decreased plasma glutamine concentration post-exercise is the main reason for the contemporary decreased immune function is based on studies showing that:

- Glutamine is important for cells in culture.
- Cells of the immune system have a high capacity for glutamine oxidation.
- Glutamine addition *in vitro* enhances lymphocyte proliferation and LAK cell activity and increases the production of some T-cell derived cytokines.

Furthermore, studies in animals have shown a beneficial effect of glutamine addition to total parenteral nutrition resulting in:

- less efflux of glutamine from skeletal muscles
- improved nitrogen balance
- less villus atrophy in the gut

Several studies have tried to link the changes in the immune system induced by exercise or other stress situations to changes in plasma glutamine concentration.[5,21,22,30,53]

The *in vitro* studies clearly show that glutamine enhances the mitogen-stimulated response in a concentration-dependent manner with optimal proliferation at glutamine concentrations between 100 and 600 mM.[39] The *in vivo* decrease in plasma glutamine concentration in relation to exercise is approximately 100 mM, dependent on the type and duration of the exercise, and the lowest plasma glutamine concentration reported in the literature in relation to catabolic conditions is 200 mM measured after major burns. Results from the *in vitro* studies show that the glutamine concentration has to be less than 100 mM to observe a decreased proliferation response.[18,39] If this is compared with the results from the *in vivo* studies,[23,25] with relatively small decreases (10–20 %) in plasma glutamine concentration, it is unlikely that glutamine supplementation and restoration of the plasma glutamine concentration would influence the proliferation response and LAK-cell activity. It can, however, not be excluded that glutamine concentrations decline more in other tissues than in the blood compartment.

The fact that glutamine supplementation does not restore post-exercise impairment of various immune functions is not likely to be based on a discrepancy between results as such, but is explained by the fact that the concentration of glutamine after exercise is not suppressed to levels inducing decrease of immune function *in vitro*. However, it cannot be excluded that *in vivo,* the metabolism of glutamine in the lymphocytes is influenced by exercise-induced changes in, e.g., the hormonal environment. It remains to be shown if glutamine supplementation has any effect on the immune system in subjects with resting chronic low plasma glutamine concentrations.

A weak point in the "glutamine hypothesis" in regard to the *in vitro* influence of glutamine is that when glutamine at a concentration identical to the lowest plasma glutamine concentration obtained post-exercise (300–400 mM) is added to lymphocytes, these will function equally as well as when glutamine is added at a concentration identical to the resting level (600 mM). Glutamine supplementation studies from our laboratory as well as other studies have shown that maintenance of the plasma glutamine concentration does not influence the exercise-induced changes in lymphocyte proliferation, LAK-cell activity, or distribution of lymphocytes. Therefore, until now the available data on humans do not support the contention that post-exercise decline in plasma-glutamine concentration plays a major mechanistic role in post-exercise immune impairment.

ACKNOWLEDGMENT

The research for this chapter was supported by The National Research Foundation grant #504-14.

REFERENCES

1. Newsholme, P., Gordon, S., and Newsholme, E.A., Rates of utilization and fates of glucose, glutamine, pyruvate, fatty acids and ketone bodies by mouse macrophages. *Biochem.J.*, 242, 631., 1987.
2. Ardawi, M.S. and Newsholme, E.A., Glutamine metabolism in lymphocytes of the rat. *Biochem. J.*, 212, 835, 1983.
3. Newsholme, E.A., Biochemical mechanisms to explain immunosuppression in well-trained and overtrained athletes. *Int. J. Sports Med.*, 15, S142, 1994.
4. Ardawi, M.S. and Newsholme, E.A., Intracellular localization and properties of phosphate-dependent glutaminase in rat mesenteric lymph nodes. *Biochem. J.*, 217, 289, 1984.
5. Newsholme, E.A., Psychoimmunology and cellular nutrition: an alternative hypothesis [editorial]. *Biol. Psychiatry*, 27, 1, 1990.
6. Newsholme, E.A., Newsholme, P., Curi, R., Challoner, E., and Ardawi, M.S.M., A role for muscle in the immune system and its importance in surgery, trauma, sepsis, and burns. *Nutrition*, 4, 261, 1990.
7. Hoffman-Goetz, L. and Pedersen, B.K., Exercise and the immune system: a model of the stress response? *Immunol. Today*, 15, 382, 1994.
8. Mackinnon, L.T., Chick, T.W., van As, A., and Tomasi, T.B., The effect of exercise on secretory and natural immunity. *Adv. Exp. Med. Biol.*, 216A, 869, 1987.
9. Nieman, D.C., Exercise, infection, and immunity. *Int. J. Sports Med.*, 15 Suppl 3, S131-S141, 1994.
10. Friman, G. and Ilback, N.G., Exercise and infection—interaction, risks, and benefits. *Scand. J. Med. Sci. Sports*, 2, 177, 1992.
11. Rose, W.C., The nutritive significance of the amino acids. *Physiol. Rev.*, 18, 109, 1938.
12. Eagle, H. *Science*, 501, 1955.
13. Eagle, H. *J. Biol. Chem.*,607, 1955.

14. Rennie, M.J., Edwards, R.H.T., Krywawych, S., Davies, C.T., Halliday, D., and Waterlow, J.C., Effect of exercise on protein turnover in man. *Clin. Sci.*, 61, 639, 1981.
15. Windmueller, H.G. and Spaeth, A.E. *J. Biol. Chem.*, 5070, 1974.
16. Kovacevic, Z. and McGivan, J.D., Mitochondrial metabolism of glutamine and glutamate and its physiological significance. *Physiol. Rev.*, 63, 547, 1983.
17. Ardawi, M.S. and Newsholme, E.A., Maximum activities of some enzymes of glycolysis, the tricarboxylic acid cycle and ketone-body and glutamine utilization pathways in lymphocytes of the rat. *Biochem. J.*, 208, 743, 1982.
18. Rohde, T., MacLean, D.A., and Pedersen, B.K., Glutamine, lymphocyte proliferation and cytokine production. *Scand. J. Immunol.*, (in press).
19. McKeehan, W.L,. Glycolysis, glutaminolysis and cell proliferation. *Cell Biol. Int. Rep.*, 6, 635, 1982.
20. Smith, R.J., Glutamine metabolism and its physiologic importance. *JPEN. J. Parenter. Enteral. Nutr.*, 14, 40S, 1990.
21. Keast, D., Arstein, D., Harper, W., Fry, R.W., and Morton, A.R., Depression of plasma glutamine concentration after exercise stress and its possible influence on the immune system. *Med. J. Aust.*, 162, 15, 1995.
22. Parry Billings, M., Budgett, R., Koutedakis, Y., Blomstrand, E., Brooks, S., Williams, C., Calder, P.C., Pilling, S., Baigrie, R., and Newsholme, E.A. Plasma amino acid concentrations in the overtraining syndrome: possible effects on the immune system. *Med. Sci. Sports Exerc.*, 24, 1353, 1992.
23. Rohde, T., Asp, S., MacLean, D.A., and Pedersen, B.K., Competitive sustained exercise in humans, lymphokine-activated killer cell activity, and glutamine — an intervention study. *Eur. J. Appl.Physiol.*, 78, 448, 1998.
24. Rohde, T., MacLean, D.A., Hartkopp, A., and Pedersen, B.K., The immune system and serum glutamine during a triathlon. *Eur. J. Appl. Physiol.*, 74, 428, 1996.
25. Rohde, T., MacLean, D., and Pedersen, B.K., Effect of glutamine on changes in the immune system induced by repeated exercise. *Med. Sci. Sports Exerc.*, 30, 856, 1998.
26. Lehmann, M., Huonker, M., Dimeo, F., Heinz, N., Gastmann, U., Treis, N., Steinackcr, J.M., Keul, J., Kajewski, R., and Haussinger, D., Serum amino acid concentrations in nine athletes before and after the 1993 Colmar ultra triathlon. *Int. J. Sports Med.*, 16, 155, 1995.
27. Zanker, C.L., Swaine, I.L., Castell, L.M., and Newsholme, E.A., Responses of glutamine, free tryptophan and branched-chain amino acids to prolonged exercise after a regime designed to reduce muscle glycogen. *Eur. J. Appl. Physiol.*, 75, 543, 1997.
28. Askanazi, J., Furst, P., Michelsen, C.B., Elwyn, D.H., Vinnars, E., Gump, F.E., Stinchfield, F.E., and Kinney, J.E., Muscle and plasma amino acids after injury; hypocaloric glucose vs. amino acid infusion. *Ann. Surg.*, 191, 465, 1980.
29. Essen, P., Wernerman, J., Sonnenfeld, T., Thunell, S., and Vinnars, E., Free amino acids in plasma and muscle during 24 hours post-operatively — a descriptive study. *Clin. Physiol.*, 12, 163, 1992.
30. Parry Billings, M., Evans, J., Calder, P.C., and Newsholme, E.A., Does glutamine contribute to immunosuppression after major burns? *Lancet*, 336, 523, 1990.
31. Hiscock, N. and Mackinnon, L.T., A comparison of plasma glutamine concentration in athletes from different sports. *Med. Sci. Sports Exerc.*,30, 1693, 1998.
32. Rowbottom, D.G., Keast, D., Garcia-Webb, P., and Morton, A.R., Training adaptation and biological changes among well-trained male triathletes. *Med. Sci. Sports Exerc.*,29, 1233, 1997.
33. Rowbottom, D.G., Keast, D., and Morton, A.R., The emerging role of glutamine as an indicator of exercise stress and overtraining. *Sports Med.*, 21, 80, 1996.

34. Walsh, N.P., Blannin, A.K., Robson, P.J., and Gleeson, M., Glutamine, exercise and immune function. Links and possible mechanisms. *Sports Med.*, 26, 177, 1998.

35. Mackinnon, L.T. and Hooper, S.L., Plasma glutamine and upper respiratory tract infection during intensified training in swimmers. *Med. Sci. Sports Exerc.*, 28, 285, 1996.

36. Reitzer, L.J., Wice, B.M., and Kennell, D., Evidence that glutamine, not sugar, is the major energy source for cultured HeLa cells. *J. Biol. Chem.*, 254, 2669, 1979.

37. Zielke, H.R., Ozand, P.T., Tildon, J.T., Sevdalian, D.A., and Cornblath, M., Reciprocal regulation of glucose and glutamine utilization by cultured human diploid fibroblasts. *J.Cell Physiol.*, 95, 41, 1978.

38. Crawford, J. and Cohen, H.J., The essential role of L-glutamine in lymphocyte differentiation in vitro. *J.Cell Physiol.*, 124, 275, 1985.

39. Rohde, T., Ullum, H., Palmo, J., Halkjaer Kristensen, J., Newsholme, E.A., and Pedersen, B.K., Effects of glutamine on the immune system- influence of muscular exercise and HIV infection. *J. Appl. Physiol.*, 79, 146, 1995.

40. Wallace, C. and Keast, D., Glutamine and macrophage function. *Metabolism*, 41, 1016, 1992.

41. Calder, P.C. and Newsholme, E.A., Glutamine promotes interleukin-2 production by concanavalian A-stimulated lymphocytes. *Proc. Nutr. Soc.*, 51, 105A, 1992.

42. Juretic, A., Spagnoli, G.C., Horig, H., Rabst, R., von Bremen, K., and Harder, F., Glutamine requirements in the generation of lymphokine-activated killer cells. *Clin. Nutr.*, 13, 42, 1994.

43. Fahr, M.J., Kornbluth, J., Blossom, S., Schaeffer, R., and Klimberg, V.S., Glutamine enhances immunoregulation of tumour growth. *J. Parenter. Enteral. Nutr.*, 18, 471, 1994.

44. Scheltinga, M.R., Young, L.S., Benfell, K., Bye, R.L., Ziegler, T.R., Santos, A.A., Antin, J.H., Schloerb, P.R., and Wilmore, D.W., Glutamine-enriched intravenous feedings attenuate extracellular fluid expansion after a standard stress. *Am. Surg.*, 214, 385, 1991.

45. Burke, D.J., Alverdy, J.C., Aoys, E., and Moss, G.S., Glutamine-supplemented total parenteral nutrition improves gut immune function. *Arch. Surg.*, 124, 1396, 1989.

46. Yoshida, S., Yonoki, T., Aoyagi, K., Ohta, J., Ishibashi, N., and Noake, T. Effect of glutamine supplement and hepatectomy on DNA and protein synthesis in the remnant liver. *J. Surg. Res*, 59, 475, 1995.

47. Yoshida, S., Yamasaki, K., Kaibara, A., Mizote, H., and Takegawa, T., Glutamine (Gln) supplementation in septic rats. *Nippon. Geka. Gakkai. Zasshi.*, 94, 1078, 1993.

48. Buchman, A.L., Mestecky, A., Moukarzel, A., and Ament, M.E., Intestinal immune function is unaffected by parenteral nutrition in man. *J. Am. Coll. Nutr.*, 14, 656, 1995.

49. Buchman, A.L., Moukarzel, A.A., Bhuta, S., Belle, M., Ament, M.E., and Eckert, C.D., Parenteral nutrition is associated with intestinal morphologic and functional changes in humans. *J. Parenter. Enteral. Nutr.*, 19, 453, 1995.

50. Shewchuk, L.D., Baracos, V.E., and Field, C.J., Dietary L-glutamine does not improve lyphocyte metabolism or function in exercise-trained rats. *Med. Sci. Sports Exerc.*, 29, 474, 1997.

51. Koyama, K., Kaya, M., Tsujita, J., and Hori, S., Effects of decreased plasma glutamine concentrations on peripheral lymphocyte proliferation in rats. *Eur. J. Appl. Physiol*, 77, 25, 1998.

52. Hack, V., Weiss, C., Friedmann, B., Suttner, S., Schykowski, M., and Erbe, N., Decreased plasma glutamine level and CD4+ T cell number in response to 8 wk of anaerobic training. *Am. J. Physiol.*, 272, E788-E795, 1997.

53. Castell, L.M., Poortmans, J.R., and Newsholme, E.A., Does glutamine have a role in reducing infections in athletes? *Eur. J. Appl. Physiol.*, 73, 488, 1996.
54. Castell, L.M., Poortmans, J.R., Leclercq, R., Brasseur, M., Duchateau, J., and Newsholme, E.A., Some aspects of the acute phase response after a marathon race, and the effects of glutamine supplementation. *Eur. J. Appl. Physiol.*, 75, 47, 1997.

CHAPTER 6

Vitamins, Immunity, and Infection Risk in Athletes

Edith M. Peters

CONTENTS

1-8493-0741-4/00/$0.00+$.50
© 2000 by CRC Press LLC

6.1 INTRODUCTION

Success in elite sport is dependent on the maintenance of peak physiological function. Athletes must endure extreme levels of physical and psychological stress during repeated cycles of exhaustive exercise in both training and during competition. Despite many reports of increased risk of infection and reduced ability to perform during periods of heavy training and after intense competitive events,[1-2] evidence of a reduction of infection risk has also been reported in well-trained athletes.[3] Herein lies the apparent paradox of exercise and infection risk.

On the one hand, an increase in fitness level resulting from frequent, regular exercise training at moderate intensity may have a protective effect and has been associated with a lower infection incidence.[4] On the other, athletes may be at increased risk of infection purely by virtue of the greater presence of pathological microorganisms in the physical environment in which they are practicing their sport;[5] their greater vulnerability to sustaining abrasions, contusions, and a variety of soft-tissue injury;[6] and, in the event of maximal endurance activities, enhanced ventilatory rates and volumes over prolonged periods might result in increased intake of potential pathogens causing localized mechanical trauma and inflammatory damage to the sensitive epithelial tissues of the upper respiratory tract.[7] The changed systemic endocrine–cytokine milieu is also thought to contribute to lowered resistance and greater predisposition to infection.[8]

Nutritional consideration is inextricably linked to the preparation and care of elite athletes. As it has now been established that deficiencies of single micronutrients may affect immunocompetence,[9] the role of vitamins is receiving greater prominence in research *foci*. In this chapter, the findings of recent dietary surveys that have focused on vitamin intake in elite sportspersons, the evidence in support of altered infection risk following prolonged periods of heavy exertion and intensive training regimes, and the possible benefits or adverse effects of a positive vitamin and pro-vitamin status will be reviewed.

6.2 VITAMIN INTAKE PRACTICES OF ELITE ATHLETES

Defined as organic compounds that are needed in very small quantities in the diet, vitamins are essential for specific metabolic reactions in the body and to promote normal growth and development. With the exception of vitamin D, which can be synthesized in the presence of sunlight, vitamin K, and small quantities of selected B-vitamins that can be produced by the micro-flora of the gastrointestinal tract, vitamins are not produced by the human body and must be consumed in the diet.[10] Although not reported to directly contribute toward energy supply, they do play an important role in regulating metabolism; a deficiency of certain of the B-group that act as co-factors of enzymes in carbohydrate (e.g. niacin, vitamin B_6, thiamine), fat (e.g., ribo-flavin, thiamine, pantothenate, biotin) and protein (vitamin B_6) metabolism results in premature fatigue and inability to maintain a heavy athletic training program, whereas others play a role in hematopoiesis (viz. folate, vitamin B_{12}) or assist in the formation of bones, connective tissue, and cartilage (e.g., vitamins C, D).[11]

Table 6.1 Cross-Sectional Studies on Physically Active Individuals Reporting Vitamin Intakes

	Subjects	Vitamin Intake Below RDA*	Vitamin Intake Above 5x RDA*
Cohen at al., 1985[19]	Professional ballet dancers (n=22)	Vit B_6, B_{12}, folate, pantothenate, biotin	Vit B_1, B_2
Benson et al., 1985[20]	Ballet dancers (n=92)	Vit B_6# folate#	–
Loosi et al., 1986[21]	Competitive adolescent female gymnasts (n=97)	Vit B_6, B_{12}, folate	–
Burke and Read, 1987[22]	Elite Australian athletes	–	–
Nieman et al., 1989[23]	Marathoners (n=347)	Vit B_{12}	–
Van Erp Baart et al., 1989[24]	Elite endurance (n=222)	Vit B_1(PC), B_6, C(S)	–
	Elite strength (n=103)	Vit A(FG, FBB), B_6 (A),C(FG)	–
	Elite Team (n=84)	Vit B_6, C(H)	–
Singh et al., 1993[25]	Ultramarathoners (n=17)	–	
Niekamp, 1995[26]	Trained male cross-country runners (n=12)	–	–
Peters and Goetzske, 1997[27]**	Ultramarathoners (n=173) • Training diets	Vit D	Vit B_2, B_6, B_{12}, C Vit B_2, B_6, B_{12}, C
	• Pre-race diets	Vit D	
Govender, 1998[28]**	Marathoners (n=56) • Whites (n=25) • Indians (n=31)		

*RDA: Recommended Daily Allowances[18]; **Combined dietary intake in food and supplements; #>70% consumed less than two-thirds of RDA; FG: female gymnasts; FBB: female body builders; PC: professional cyclists; S: swimmers; H: handball players.

Ideally, athletes should obtain all their nutrients from food. A well-balanced diet including foods from each of the five food groups should provide adequate amounts of all 13 essential vitamins.[12] It is argued that as the total energy intake of most athletes exceeds that of sedentary non-athletes, a greater number and variety of vitamins should be available to the athlete through dietary intake.[12–13] Unfortunately, dietary surveys indicate that athletes do, however, not always consume a well-balanced diet.

Elite athletes are at high risk of developing nutrient deficiencies due to the grueling demands of training. A combination of high turnover, a loss of some nutrients and limited time for food preparation are contributing factors.[14,15] The first two comprehensive reports of the actual dietary intakes of athletes published in 1981[15,16] reported inappropriate macronutrient composition of the diets with too great a fat and protein component, and in the study of Barry et al.,[15] this was coupled with sub-optimal intakes of thiamine, niacin, iron, and folate well below the recommended daily requirements[17] in the female athletes. The results of subsequent dietary surveys performed on elite endurance athletes since 1985 are presented in Table 6.1.

It is of interest that, besides the low vitamin D intakes in South African runners,[27,28] deficient as well as excess intakes are fairly consistent for water-soluble vitamins, with the exception of vitamin A in the Dutch elite strength athletes.[24] Although it is well accepted that additional intake of these vitamins does not contribute to enhanced performance,[29,30] the effect of the high total intake of vitamin C and a number of the vitamin B group in the recent study on ultramarathoners, and of the deficient intakes of a variety of water-soluble vitamins on immune function will be addressed in this chapter. It is, however, first necessary to examine the effect of physical activity alone on immune function as it manifests in the incidence of clinical infection.

6.3 ALTERED INFECTION RISK FOLLOWING PHYSICAL EXERTION: THE EXERCISE PARADOX

The paradoxical relationship between exercise and upper respiratory infection (URTI) risk that has been modeled as a "J"-shaped curve[31] is well documented. Whereas regular training at moderate intensity and quantity over a prolonged period is postulated to reduce the risk of infection below that of a sedentary individual and has apparent chronic immunomodulatory effects, once a critical threshold is reached, the more strenuous, prolonged, and/or frequent the exercise, the greater the risk of infection and lower immunosurveillance (Figure 6.1). We will discuss some of the evidence in support of this apparently conflicting relationship between exercise and infection risk.

6.3.1 Exercise as Panacea for Illness?

Anecdotal reports of increased resistance to infection in well-trained endurance athletes abound. But, at present, very limited data suggest an enhancement of resistance to infections from regular moderate exercise training.

Few longitudinal studies have been designed specifically to consider the chronic effects of repeated bouts of exercise on the incidence of URTI. A survey of the illness patterns of a cohort of 530 male and female runners over a period of 12 months[33] revealed a lower average number of self-reported infectious episodes per runner than those reported in three previous studies of non-athletic individuals.[34–37] Controlling for various confounding variables, the lowest odds ratio for respiratory infection was found among those running less than 16 km per week and more than doubled for those running more than 27 km per week.[33]

This finding of a reduction of infection risk following a prolonged session of regular exercise of moderate intensity and volume is, however, not confirmed by all

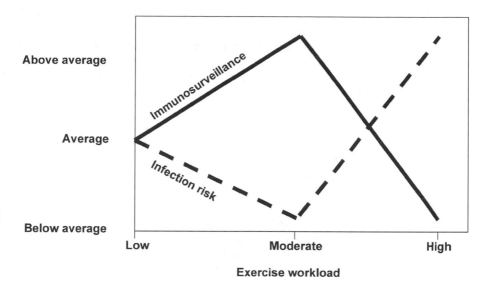

Figure 6.1   The paradoxical relationship between exercise workload, risk of URTI, and immunosurvelllance in athletes. (Adapted from Nieman.[32])

studies. It is possible that training volume is only one variable that significantly affects infection risk[4] and that a range of dietary, psychological, and environmental factors could explain the absence of a relationship between training intensity/volume and incidence of infection in these studies.[38–41]

Morc-recent, well-controlled studies on circulating immune variables provide limited, yet consistent supportive evidence in favor of a possible protective effect to be obtained from exercise of moderate intensity.[3, 42–44] A 15-week exercise training program comprising five 45-min sessions/wk[-1] of brisk walking at 60% hcart-rate reserve in 36 mildly obese, sedentary women[3, 42–44] resulted in a significant reduction in symptoms of URTI with almost 50% of the number of days with symptoms in exercisers than the sedentary control group. This was accompanied by decreases in percentage and number of total lymphocytes and T cell number [3, 44] and a 20% increase in serum immunoglobin levels.[45] In a second 12-week study,[46] the lowest incidence (8%) of URTI symptoms was reported in a group of highly conditioned elderly female subjects who exercised moderately each day for about 1.5 hr, as compared with a group exercising for only 40 min five times per week and a sedentary control group, suggesting that frequency of exercise may also affect immunosurveillance.

6.3.2 Increased Infection Risk

The early notion of an apparently greater risk of infection following single bouts of severe exertion, and subsequent references to the association between altered infection risk and exercise training was also based only on anecdotal reports from coaches and sports physicians.[47–49] In 1975, Ryan[50] concluded that "combined with accompanying secondary infections and related problems, URTIs cause more dis-ability among athletes than all other diseases combined." This was later confirmed by an extensive study on a group of 310 elite Swedish cross-country skiers over 12 months,[52] in which it was found that infectious disease, in particular, URTI, was the most commonly reported reason for absence from training in the athletes surveyed.

The first prospective report of an epidemiological study revealing a higher incidence of URTI following intensive exercise, compared with the incidence in matched controls who did not run,[52] was published in 1983. Sore throats, nasal symptoms, cough, and fever in runners were significantly higher (p<0.005) during the fortnight following a 56-km ultramarathon running event. Symptoms of URTI occurred in 47% of the runners who completed the race in less than 4 h, compared with 19% of those finishing the race in between 5 h 30 min and 6h, and 15.3% in the non-running members of their households during the same period. The duration of the symptoms suggested that they were not trivial in origin. This finding of an increased incidence of URTI during the post-race fortnight was confirmed when the same study design was repeated on another group of 104 participants in a 56-km ultramarathon that took place at 1800 m above sea-level [53] and by the findings of a large-scale study performed on 2311 marathon runners competing in a standard marathon (42 km) in Los Angeles.[54] Despite the shorter distance of this race, 12.9% of the 1828 runners who did not report infectious episodes before the race docu-mented an infection during the first 7 days following the marathon vs. 2.2% in controls (well-trained non-participating runners). Controlling for important demo-graphic and training data by using logistic regression, it was determined that the odds were 6 to 1 in favor of sickness for the marathoners when compared with the non-participating control runners. Other interesting results of this extensive work included the finding that the odds of infection risk in the runners covering more than 96 km/wk were double those in runners completing less than 32 km/wk in training. A significant increase in the odds ratio occurred only once the runners had exceeded 60 km/wk in training.

These early studies indicating an increased infection risk associated with exhaus-tive exercise were, however, not limited to acute exposure to single bouts of pro-longed exercise. In 1987, over a 12-month period, in a group of 44 elite Danish orienteers and 44 non-athletes, it was reported that not only was the incidence, but also the duration, of URTI greater in the elite athletes.[55] Together with the previously described longitudinal study conducted on a cohort of 530 marathoners over 12 months,[33] these findings have been supported by numerous smaller studies[56-62] that confirmed the link of infection risk to quantity, intensity, and frequency of training, and the premise that not only acute exposure to exhaustive exercise, but also over-training and undertraining[59-62] result in an increased infection risk in athletes follow-ing exhaustive prolonged exercise.

These data are supported by recent evidence of the immune profile of well-conditioned elite athletes that do suggest a possible down-regulation of the immune system in the case of excessive training.[62-65] Lower neutrophil oxidative capacity during a 12-week period of intensive training prior to competition;[63] significantly lower salivary IgA levels in "stale," overtrained as compared with those of well-trained, elite Australian swimmers over a 6-month period;[65] and a downward trend in serum and salivary IgA levels of pre- and post-exercise in elite swimmers monitored over a 7-month period[64] suggest that aspects of both systemic and mucosal immunity may be suppressed during prolonged periods of intensive training. A strong inverse relationship between mean pre-training salivary IgA levels and the incidence of URTI (p=0.02) have supported the use of salivary IgA levels as most predictive for athletes at risk of infection.[66]

Current available evidence thus supports the paradoxical relationship depicted in the J-shaped curve.[31] Excessive physical activity, whether it be one acute, prolonged, exhaustive exposure — particularly in the untrained individual — or too frequent, regular heavy training, may lower resistance to infection. It would appear that any form of overexertion that exceeds a critical threshold level invites infection.

6.3.3 Etiology of Increased Infection Risk

At this stage, it is not known what the physiological basis of the above-described increased susceptibility to infection among athletes is — decreased proliferative response of the lymphocytes, depression of the immune system by corticosteroids produced under physical stress, or harm done to the immune system by oxygen radicals generated during heavy exercise are among the possible explanations.[67]

It is well accepted that symptoms of infection can be triggered by infective, inflammatory, or allergic factors. A number of reviews [67–72] have outlined that acute prolonged exercise bouts result in a immunological response that appears to mimic the body's response to infection: a rise in core body temperature,[73] plasma levels of acute phase proteins and cytokines[71–72] accompanied by leukocytosis,[67] lymphopenia,[69] monocytosis,[69] and suppressed neutrophil activity.[74] Pederson and Ullum[75] have identified the existence of an "open window" during the first 6–20 hours following strenuous exertion. During this transient post-exercise period, lymphocyte numbers, NK activity, complement, and IgA levels drop.[75] These Danish researchers contend that it is during this transient "open window" period that the athlete is most vulnerable to infection; that microbacterial agents can invade the host and infections easily develop.[75] A strong association between signs of exercise-induced immunosupression and actual clinical manifestation in the form of infection symptoms, has, however, not yet been shown.[67] Pyne and Gleeson[63] point out that the transient and modest nature of the observed changes might be indicative of a "self-modulating immune cell network capable of homeostatic regulation." This perhaps accounts for the rapid post-exercise recovery of most markers of immune response.

Exercise-induced infection, and in particular URTI, can thus, at this stage, not be solely attributed to infectious origins. During prolonged endurance exercise, increased ventilatory rates and volumes with actual damage to sensitive mucous membranes in the respiratory tract and an inflammatory response at the sites of muscle cell damage have been linked to the development of an acute phase reaction.[71, 72] Shephard[77] refers to the "active enmeshment" of the immune system in the muscle tissue repair and inflammation process and speculates that in this process, protection from URTI is compromised.

Gabriel and Kinderman[74] have recently added an additional perspective. They emphasize an important difference between the apparent exercise-induced acute-phase protein response and that induced by a bacterial infection; that the leukocytosis following strenuous exercise is associated with impaired oxidative burst activity and suppressed defense mechanisms, whereas the leukocytosis present in a bacterial infection is accompanied by primed cells, enhanced neutrophil function and stimulated defense mechanisms.

It is well known that indomethacin decreases *in vitro* release of prostaglandin E_2 from mononuclear cells and restores suppressed post-exercise neutrophil chemiluminescence and NK cell activity.[78] A recent work on URTI following participation in the 1996 Two Oceans Ultramarathon[79] showed that administration of a different topical anti-inflammatory, anti-bacterial spray, Fusafungine, resulted in an actual lowering of the incidence of URTI in 48 participants when compared with an equal number of runners receiving a placebo during the 9 days following the event.

The most recent state of the knowledge thus appears to support that increased infection risk may indeed be caused by the interaction of a combination of pro-infective and pro-inflammatory responses that are modulated by the presence of physical, psychological, and environmental stresses placed on the athlete engaging in elite endurance sport.

6.4 VITAMINS, THE IMMUNE RESPONSE, AND INFECTION RISK

Vitamins have been described as interacting with the immune system in two fundamental ways. First, rapid protein synthesis and proliferation of immuno-competent cells such as B-lymphocytes are dependent on nutrient supply, which is modulated by the presence of sufficient vitamins.[80] In addition, the antioxidant vitamins (provitamins, carotenoids, and flavenoids), fulfill an additional immuno-modulatory role by preventing tissue damage caused by oxidants derived from stimulation of the immune system.[81] Whereas deficiency of some vitamins may result in dysfunction of the acquired immune components, decreased intake of the antioxidant vitamins may result in the accumulation of phagocyte-derived oxidants and contribute to accelerated onset of degenerative disease resulting from the oxidative damage.[82]

Despite the well described association of antioxidant function with lowered DNA damage, reduced lipid peroxidation and diminished *in vitro* malignant transformation, and the premise that peak operation of the cellular host immune responses is dependent on adequate availability of vitamins to the various immunocompetent cells,[80] only a prolonged and severe deficiency is thought to manifest with an actual increase in infectious episodes. Anderson[82] attributes this to the inherent reserve capacity of these cellular immune components.

It is, in particular, vitamins A, several of the B vitamins (especially vitamin B_6), vitamin C, vitamin D, vitamin E, and β-carotene for which convincing evidence of beneficial immunomodulatory effects in humans have been described and that play an active role in promoting optimum protective host immune responses.[82] Of additional interest to the athletic individual are certain provitamins and other categories of the carotenoid and flavenoid groups.[10]

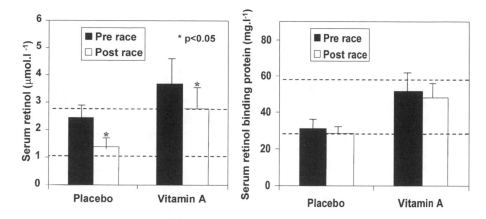

Figure 6.2 Pre- and post-race serum retinol and serum retinol-binding protein levels in runners receiving vitamin A and placebo supplementation prior to the 1991 Comrades Marathon. (Adapted from Peters et al.[59])

6.4.1 Vitamin A

In 1968, Scrimshaw et al.[83] stated that "no nutritional deficiency in the animal kingdom is more consistently synergistic with infection than that of vitamin A." They listed 50 studies in support of this contention. Although the increased risk of infection associated with a deficiency of this "anti-infective vitamin"[80] is accompanied by compromised antibody production (especially those of the IgG_1 and IgG_3 subclasses), reduced levels of natural-killer cells and loss of integrity in various epithelial surfaces including those of the respiratory tract,[85, 86] a protective effect of vitamin A supplementation has, primarily, been shown in vitamin A-deficient or marginally deficient patients.[85-87] Not only have many studies shown that supplementing vitamin A in hyporetinemic children results in increases in serum concentrations of measles IgG antibody[87] and reduces the occurrence and severity of measles,[85, 86] but a reduced incidence of mortality in children hospitalized with this infectious disease has also been reported.[87]

Few studies have, however, described a significant lowering of post-event infection risk in healthy active individuals. In a double-blind, placebo-controlled study in which ultramarathon runners received 50,000 IU vitamin A per day,[59] a 3-week period of supplementation of this vitamin did not result in a statistically significant reduction in post-race URTI incidence. Of additional interest was the fact that although both serum retinol and serum retinol-binding protein dropped significantly as a result of participation in the 88-km race, they did not drop to deficient levels (Figure 6.2). It was concluded that lack of difference in post-race infection incidence could possibly be attributed to the small groups from whom compliance was obtained in the study (n=36) and to the weak antioxidant properties of vitamin A. In addition, the possibility of the benefits of vitamin A supplementation applying only to hyporetinemic individuals is an area that requires further investigation.

6.4.2 B-Vitamins

As the B-vitamins play an important role as co-enzymes in the metabolism of lipids, carbohydrates, proteins, and nucleic acids, they possibly act as controlling factors in the active or rapidly proliferating effector cells of the immune system. As early as 1921 Cramer et al.[88] first reported an association between vitamin B deficiencies and atrophy of lymphoid tissues and lymphopenia in rats. vitamin B_6, folate, and pantothenate deficiencies have been linked to impaired immune function and impaired synthesis of antibodies.[89] Of these, it is vitamin B_6 that may be of specific interest to the exercising individual.

6.4.2.1 Vitamin B_6

This is a collective term for the metabolically and functionally related pyrodoxines and their phosphorylated forms. Pyridoxal-5-phosphate is a co-enzyme form of vitamin B_6, which, in addition to being bound to muscle glycogen phosphorylase, is particularly active in the metabolism of amino acids and proteins. As this includes nucleotide and protein synthesis, significant impact of this vitamin on immune responses has been reported.[90]

Vitamin B_6 is required for the development and function of the T-lymphocytes, which, in turn, control antibody production by the B lymphocytes. Severe deficiency of this vitamin in animals has provided consistent evidence of down-regulation of both cell-mediated and humoral immunity, which include a markedly diminished antibody response; numerous studies have also confirmed that a deficiency in the elderly is associated with a reduction in the number and function of circulating T-lymphocytes.[90,91]

Investigating the effects of a vitamin B_6 depletion–repletion regimen in healthy elderly adults,[91] it was found that vitamin B_6 depletion significantly decreased the percentage and total number of lymphocytes, as well as the mitogenic responses of peripheral blood lymphocytes to T- and B-cell mitogens. These parameters returned to baseline levels when physiological levels of vitamin B_6 (1.90 mg/d for women, 2.88 mg/d) for men were provided. It was concluded that older adults may require higher amounts of this vitamin than is currently recommended.[91]

This increased vitamin B_6 intake may also be required in the event of the consumption of high-protein diets. Bodybuilders and other sportsmen relying on these diets would therefore be groups at risk of developing marginal deficiencies of pyridoxine. Although it has been found that marathon running results in a mean loss of about 1 mg vitamin B_6,[92] no study has to date examined the relationships among high-intensity or resistive exercise, immunocompetence, and vitamin B_6 status. This would be an interesting area of investigation.

6.4.3 Vitamin D

Exposure to the active metabolite of vitamin D_3, 1,25-dihydroxy vitamin D_3 has been reported to both augment the antimycobacterial activity of human monocytes[93] and mediate the action of this agent with the vitamin D receptor, modulating the activity of genes that regulate cell growth and differentiation.[94] Although hypovita-minosis D has been shown to compromise host defenses against selected bacteria[93] and predispose to the progression of carcinomas of the breast, prostate and colon,[90] the results of low dietary vitamin D intake by athletes[27,28] must be seen in the light of the difficulties in accurately quantitating the vitamin D contents of foods and sunlight-induced endogenous production of vitamin D_3 derivatives. Together with the possible consumption of vitamin D-fortified foods and the relatively high order of toxicity of this vitamin,[10] these factors mitigate against the indiscriminate use of vitamin D supplements by athletes. Vitamin D toxicity has been shown to be asso-ciated with hypercalcaemia, hypercalciuria, bone demineralization and calcification of various soft tissues, including those in the heart, kidneys, and lungs.[94]

6.4.4 Antioxidant Vitamins and Provitamins

Whereas the major function of vitamins has classically been described as their role in facilitating energy supply, their function as scavengers of oxygen-derived free radicals was only identified in the 1980s and is today seen as a second major function of these micronutrients.[80] In particular, the vitamin C-, E-, β-carotene (precursor of vitamin A)- and other nonvitamin A-forming carotenoids, play an important role in supplementing the intracellular antioxidant enzymes (e.g. glu-tathione peroxidase, superoxide dismutase).[95] Considering the prolonged elevation in oxidative metabolism that may be increased more than 8–10 fold during endurance exercise, and the fact that it has been estimated that up to 2% of oxygen consumption is converted to toxic free radicals,[96] numerous detailed accounts of the damaging effects of oxidative stress on cell membrane lipids, carbohydrates, sulphur-containing enzymes and other proteins, as well as nucleotides,[91–93] neutrophil function[98, 99] and lymphocyte apotosis[100] following exhaustive exercise may support a protective role of antioxidant micronutrients in reducing oxidative damage and thereby decreasing infection risk in athletes regularly engaged in endurance exercise.[101]

But what is the evidence in favor of a reduced infection risk in endurance athletes following antioxidant vitamin supplementation?

6.4.4.1 Beta Carotene and Other Carotenoids

Preliminary studies investigating the effect of the plant-pigment and precursor of vitamin A, β-carotene, which is known to possess strong antioxidant properties and has been shown to result in corresponding increases in human buccal mucosal cells,[102–104] blood platelets,[105] mononuclear and red blood cells[106] after only one week of supplementation, do appear to support a possible protective effect of enhanced intake. Two studies on relatively small groups of ultramarathoners[61,107] have con-firmed a reduced incidence of URTI symptoms following enhanced β-carotene intake in the 3 weeks before the race, but in both studies the protective effect obtained from consuming 18 mg and 45 mg β-carotene per day respectively, appeared to be less than obtained in the groups of runners that were supplementing with vitamin C alone (Figure 6.3).

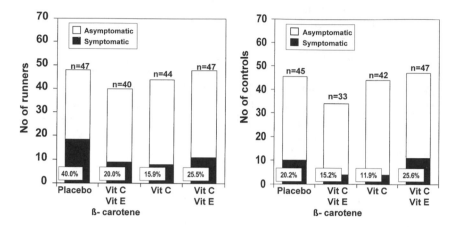

Figure 6.3   The incidence of post-race URTI symptoms in runners receiving different combinations of antioxidant supplements or placebos for 3 weeks prior to the 1993 Comrades Marathon. (Data from Peters et al.[61])

An enhancement of immune function is also known to result from an increase in circulating levels of a variety of carotenoids including β-carotene, lycopene, lutein and canthaxanthin.[105] These plant-pigment derived nutrients are frequently found in conjunction with β-carotene in fresh fruits and vegetables. Initially associated with increased time of tumor development in mice, these carotenoids possess antioxidant and singlet-quenching characteristics that are independent of pro-vitamin A activity and have been shown to reduce oxidative damage.[108] Despite this evidence, no study has yet examined the effect on immune response or infection incidence in athletes of supplementing with a broad range of carotenoids.

6.4.4.2 Vitamin C

The vitamin that has undoubtedly received the most attention in terms of its role in reducing infection risk in athletes is vitamin C.

Traditional theory holds that vitamin C has anti-infective properties; that its high concentration in leukocytes[105] is related to increases in the proliferative responses in T lymphocytes;[109–113] prevention of the suppression of neutrophil activity,[110–112] which is thought to be related to high concentrations of corticosteroids;[114] and the production of interferon and replication of viruses.[115] It is also a major biological water-soluble antioxidant that is highly effective as a scavenger of reactive oxidants in both the intracellular and extracellular compartments.[108] Its antioxidant function can be both direct, as when protecting phagocytes against auto-oxidative dysfunction[111, 112] and indirect, via its regeneration of reduced alpha-tocopherol (vitamin E).[112, 113] It is also necessary for the production of many of the hormones released during the body's stress response. These include thyroxine, adrenaline, nor-adrenaline and several other neurotransmitters.[114, 115]

Although vitamin C supplementation has repeatedly shown to result in a decrease in the severity of common cold, it has, however, not shown as consistent an effect on the incidence of the common cold.[116] Initial positive results of a meta-analysis of four placebo-controlled studies conducted by Pauling[117] were refuted by the findings of later studies and led to the widespread conviction that vitamin C has little proven effects on the incidence of the common cold.[114,115] However, recent critical reviews of these major studies have highlighted shortcomings.[118–121] Whether vitamin C actually reduces the incidence of common cold symptoms in individuals with a sedentary lifestyle thus remains unresolved.

As the highest concentrations of vitamin C are found in the adrenal glands and both adrenal as well as leukocyte vitamin C stores are rapidly depleted by various forms of stress,[109] the possibility that vitamin C supplementation may, however, boost the immune system in subjects undergoing heavy physical exertion[122] has been the focus of recent research.

In 1959, Bessel-Lorck conducted a study on 46 schoolchildren in a 9-day skiing camp and administered 1g of vitamin C per day to 20 of these children.[123] The incidence of URTI was 17% in the supplemented group as compared to 45% in those children not receiving vitamin C supplementation (n=26). Kimbarowski and Mokrow[124] later investigated former Soviet Union military recruits who had acquired influenza A infection and were presumably on a diet containing little vitamin C. Daily supplementation with 300 mg vitamin C resulted in a significantly smaller number of infected soldiers developing pneumonia than in the group not receiving vitamin C supplementation.

A major shortcoming of these two studies was, however, the possibility of bias existing between the study groups due to the failure to administer placebo control. To date, six further studies have been conducted on the incidence of URTIs in subjects under heavy physical stress (see Table 6.2).

In 1963, Ritzel conducted a carefully controlled double blind study on 279 schoolchildren in two skiing camps in the Swiss Alps.[125, 126] He administered 1g of vitamin C per day to half of these children for a period of a week and reported a substantial decrease in the number of pharyngitis, laryngitis, tonsillitis, and bronchitis episodes in the vitamin C group. In addition to a 45% decrease in the incidence of colds, there was also a 29% decrease in the mean duration of cold episodes and a 61% decrease in the total number of days of illness per person in the group receiving vitamin C. The children in this study were not only exposed to a large volume of strenuous exercise, but also to the cold weather, an added environmental stressor.[125] These findings were supported by those of Sabiston and Radomski[127] who studied 112 soldiers undergoing military training over a 2-week period in the Canadian winter and found less than half the percentage incidence of the common cold in the troops receiving 1g vitamin C per day (11%; n=56) when compared with those on placebo (25%; n=56).

In 1992, Peters et al. conducted a placebo-controlled double blind study on the effect of additional supplementation of vitamin C on 92 athletes in the South African 88-km Comrades Marathon.[59] Runners receiving an additional 600 mg of vitamin C supplementation daily reported a significantly reduced incidence of infection in the ultramarathoners during the 2-week post-race period.

Hemila[118] pooled the findings reported in these three above-mentioned placebo-controlled studies conducted following exposure to acute physical stress and supplementation over a relatively short period in relatively small subsets,[59, 125, 126] and

Table 6.2 Vitamin C Supplementation Studies Conducted on Subjects Under Heavy Physical Stress

Authors	Quantity of Daily Vitamin Supplementation	Total Daily Vit. C. Intake (mg)	Sample Size		Mode of Physical Exertion	Duration of Supplementation	%URTI Incidence
			Active Subjects	Sedentary Controls			
Bessel-Lorck, 1959[123]	Group 1: 1000 mg Group 2: none	undetermined	20 26	—	ski camp	9 days	17 45
Kimbarowski and Mokrow, 1967[124]	Group 1: 300 mg Group 2: none	300 mg & "little" in food[a]	114 112	—	Soviet military training	not reported	1.8[*a]
Ritzel, 1961[125]	Group 1: 1000 mg Group 2: placebo	undetermined	139 140	—	ski camp	1 week	12[*] 8.9[a]
Sabinston and Radomski, 1974[127]	Group 1: 1000 mg Group 2: placebo	undetermined	56 56	—	military training	2 weeks	11[*] 25
Pitt and Costrini, 1979[129]	Group 1: 2000 mg Group 2: placebo	undetermined[c]	331	—	training in marine recruits	8 weeks	27.2 26.2
Peters et al., 1993[60]	Group 1: 600 mg vit. C Group 2: placebo	1139 494	43 41	34 39	88 km run	3 weeks prior to race	33[*b] 68[b]
Peters et al., 1996[61]	Group 1: 500 mg vit C, 400 IU vit E Group 2: 600 mg vit C Group 3: 300 mg vit C, 400 IU vit E, 400 IU β-carotene Group 4: placebo	893 1004 665 585	40 44 47 47	33 41 43 45	88 km run	3 weeks prior to race	15.9 20 25.5 40.4
Moolla, 1996[107]	Group 1: 600 mg vit C Group 2: 45 mg β-carotene Group 3: placebo	undetermined	11 11	11 11	88 km run	6 weeks prior to race	30.8 41.7 68

Note: *p<0.05 when compared with incidence in unsupplemented groups; [a]subjects with influenza A who developed pneumonia; [b]symptoms lasting ≥ 1 day incuded in analysis; [c]blood vitamin C levels indicated an absence of marginal deficiency in the control group.

calculated a combined rate ratio that represented the proportion of subjects catching a common cold in the vitamin C-supplemented groups vs. the number of subjects catching a common cold in the placebo-supplemented groups. This summed ratio was 0.50.

Not included in the summed data presented by Hemila were the findings of the study of Pitt and Costrini,[128] which investigated the effect of 2 g/day of vitamin C supplementation vs. placebo during a 2-month military training camp on 674 marine recruits in South Carolina. These findings supported a reduction in the severity of the infections experienced by the military recruits with a substantially lower incidence of pneumonia in the vitamin C group, but did not confirm the findings of a lower incidence of infection in previous intervention trials. This study did, however, possess a number of differences in design from the previous studies. It is necessary to take into consideration that the subjects received supplementation only after two weeks, and were followed over a full 2-month period, which means that an adaptive response, both in terms of physical adaptation and acclimatization to the higher intake of vitamin C, may have influenced the effect of the vitamin C supplementation.[116]

Two subsequent studies on the ultramarathoners undertaken at the 1993 88-km Comrades Marathon[59, 107] confirm a lower incidence of infections following supplementation with vitamin C. In these two independent studies the effect of different combinations of vitamins C, E, and β-carotene were examined.

Peters et al.[59] randomly divided participants in the 1993 Comrades Marathon (n=178), and their matched controls (n=162) into four treatment groups receiving either 500 mg ascorbic acid (C), 500 mg vitamin C and 400 IU vitamin E (CE), 300 mg vitamin C, 300 IU vitamin E and 18mg β-carotene (CEB), or placebo (P). As runners were requested to continue with their usual habits in terms of dietary intake and the use of nutritional supplements, total vitamin C intake of the four groups was 1004, 893, 665, and 585 mg daily respectively. The study first confirmed previous findings of a lower incidence of symptoms of infection in those runners with the highest mean daily intake of vitamin C. Second, it confirmed a lower incidence of infection in the more highly endurance-trained higher runners, and higher incidence of infection in least-trained individuals. The major finding of this study, however, supports the notion that a total intake of approximately 1g of vitamin C per day for 3 weeks prior to a race does have a protective effect in ultramarathon runners in terms of reducing the URTI risk. This is considerably higher than the daily dosage of 200 mg that has been shown to be associated with accelerated clinical improvement in elderly patients hospitalized with acute respiratory infection after 4 weeks of daily supplementation.[129]

A further independent study on 47 participants in the 1993 Comrades Marathon[107] confirmed a lower incidence of infection in the 11 runners receiving 600 mg of vitamin C per day than the 11 runners receiving 45 mg of β-carotene and the 25 runners on placebo capsules. Dietary intakes of antioxidant vitamins were unfortunately not recorded in this work.

Taken together, all five placebo-controlled studies involving short-term vitamin C supplementation in subjects undergoing heavy physical exertion did confirm a reduction of the incidence of the common cold following vitamin C supplementation. Duration and magnitude of supplementation as well as physical fitness and prior dietary intake of the subjects appear to be extraneous variables that may influence the efficacy of the supplementation.

It is unlikely that the consistent collective current evidence in favor of reduced infection risk following severe physical exertion by subjects supplementing with vitamin C over a relatively short period is based on chance alone. But, when reviewing the results of these studies on distance runners collectively, two short-comings are apparent. First, the sample size used in each of these individual studies is relatively small. Furthermore, due to the publicity that early South African studies obtained regarding possible benefits to ultramarathoners of vitamin C supplementa-tion, and the fact that it was not possible, from an ethical perspective, to prevent the prospective ultramarathoners from continuing with their usual intakes of nutritional supplements, a true control group consuming low levels of vitamin C did not exist in the later studies on the ultradistance runners. It would be interesting to observe whether these findings would be replicated in a well-controlled, large-scale inter-vention study in which runners were not permitted to make use of any nutritional supplements other than the ones obtained for the purpose of the study.

6.4.4.2.1 Limited Supportive Biochemical Evidence

Phagocytes and lymphocytes can contain greater than 10 times the concentration of vitamin C in blood plasma. These, together with the high concentrations of vitamin C stored in the adrenal glands,[110] suggest the possibility of functional roles for this vitamin in the cells of the immune system during exercise. Clinical studies on exercising subjects have, however, not provided a clear indication of the mechanism by which vitamin C may have an anti-infective action.

In a randomized, double-blind, placebo-controlled study,[130] supplementation with 1000 mg of vitamin C for 8 days did not have significant effect on stress-hormone concentrations, leukocyte subsets, interleukin-6, natural-killer-cell activity, lympho-cyte proliferation, granulocyte phagocytosis or activated oxidative burst following 2.5 hours of intensive running at 75%–80% VO_{2max} (N=6). Whether immune pools of ascorbate were depleted within 2.5 hours of running on a treadmill, is, however, questionable. It would be interesting to repeat this study following a longer session of ultradistance running.

In contrast, the effect of vitamin C supplementation (1g/day) for 7 days and for 2 weeks on biomarkers of pro-oxidative (plasma thiobarbituric acid reacting sub-stances(TBARS)) and antioxidative activity oxygen radical absorbance capacity (ORAC) was determined using the TBARS:ORAC ratio to represent oxidative stress.[131] This ratio was highest (32%) following 30 min of running exercise when a placebo was given and only rose by 5.8% after one day of vitamin C supplemen-tation as opposed to 25.8% after 2 weeks of supplementation. As the increases in oxidative stress ratios, however, did not reach statistical significance, this study appeared to support only a mild tendency of biomarkers of oxidative stress to tilt the oxidative stress balance toward antioxidant activity after vitamin C supplemen-tation. Interesting is the apparently more-marked effect after an acute period of supplementation than the more-prolonged 2 weeks of supplementation. The implications of the latter finding require further investigation.

In a double-blind, placebo-controlled study, selected immune, endocrine, and cytokine parameters were investigated following participation in the 1997 88-km Comrades Marathon.[132] Significantly higher levels of vitamin C following daily supplementation with 1000 mg of vitamin C over a 10-day period were accompanied by a significant rise in plasma ascorbate and vitamin E levels (after correction for plasma volume changes) following participation in the ultramarathon. This would appear to suggest greater mobilization of ascorbate stores in subjects with lower blood concentrations during prolonged exercise, and a failure of the cell ascorbate pools to deplete in the placebo-controlled group. Neutrophil to lymphocyte ratio, lipid hydroperoxide and myloperoxidase concentration did not differ significantly between supplemented and placebo groups, yet C-reactive protein and creatine kinase levels were significantly higher in the vitamin C supplemented group, possibly indicating a pro-inflammatory effect and enhancement of the acute-phase protein response following ultradistance running.

Further reports of possible enhancement of pro-oxidative activity following supplementation with vitamin C do exist.[133–135] The theory that megadoses of vitamin C have a pro-oxidant effect was first related to its reaction with iron: that in the presence of iron, ascorbic acid converts iron stores to catalytic iron, which possesses strong pro-oxidant effects. The concern was that in the case of persons born with a gene for increased iron-absorption, high vitamin C intake, which is known to increase absorption of dietary iron,[10] can cause iron overload and the release of large amounts of catalytic iron from their body stores.[134] This is, however, only applicable to serum ferritin levels in excess of 120 ul/l.[134] As these concentrations have rarely been described in elite athletes and are not considered physiological, the possibility of an iron-associated pro-oxidant effect of vitamin C in athletes is unlikely.

The findings of a vitamin C supplementation study published in 1977[135] were that supplementing with 200 mg as well as 2000 mg per day stimulated hexose monophosphate shunt activity of resting neutrophils. Although bactericidal killing activity was not affected by the moderate dose of vitamin C supplementation, administration of a megadose resulted in a decrement of bacterial killing of the leukocytes. As the megadose of vitamin C administered was not accompanied by an increase in plasma cortisol, and circulating levels of cyclic nucleotides were not measured, these authors were unable to clarify possible mechanisms with certainty.

The most recent debate has revolved around the findings of Podmore et al.[136] that administration of 500 mg of vitamin C to healthy volunteers resulted in a decrease in 8-oxo-7,8 dihydroguanine, and an increase in 8-oxo-7,8 -dihydroadenine in lymphocyte DNA. A major criticism of this study is that intracellular vitamin C concentrations were not measured in the lymphocytes; that increasing extracellular plasma concentrate of ascorbate above 50 uM will not affect the intracellular concentration further.[137] As the study was neither placebo controlled nor double blinded, further well-designed trials are needed to resolve this question.

Caution is merited and careful consideration needs to be given to possible mechanisms by which vitamin C might exert pro-oxidative effects in vivo. Based on in vitro observations, Anderson[138] has proposed that vitamin C possesses three properties that might contribute to pro-oxidative activity *in vivo*. First, the vitamin does not scavenge H_2O_2.[112] Second, and somewhat paradoxically, vitamin C, by acting as a scavenger of HOCl, prevents auto-oxidative inactivation of NADPH-oxidase, resulting in increased production of H_2O_2 by activated phagocytes.[138] Third, vitamin C, probably by complexing with the critical heme group of catalase, inhibits the H_2O_2-neutralizing activity of this enzyme.[139] If operative *in vivo*, these pro-oxidative activities of vitamin C may predispose to H_2O_2-mediated tissue damage and genotoxicity as a result of both increased production and reactivity of this reactive oxidant.

At this stage, there is not enough concrete evidence to support the possibility of a dualistic, differential response to vitamin C supplementation. To quote Poulsen et al.,[140] "it is too soon to say whether supplemental doses of vitamin C exert pro-oxidant or mutagenic effects." The rare incidences of conflicting evidence do, however, justify the need for further research to confirm the correctness of the present assumption that megadoses of vitamin C do have beneficial antioxidant effects following exercise, and clarify the reasons for the occasional discrepant findings. Furthermore, the impact of duration and quality of the vitamin C supplementation on exercise-induced immune and inflammatory responses require determination.

6.4.4.3 Vitamin E

As a potent peroxyl radical scavenger, α-tocopherol is a chain-breaking antiox-idant that prevents the propagation of free-radical damage in the phospholipids of membranes.[141] Evidence from animal and human studies indicates that vitamin E plays an important role in the maintenance of the immune system and that even a marginal deficiency impairs immune response. In chicks, 10 times the RDA of vitamin E have been found to be immunostimulatory[142] whereas in humans, supple-mentation of healthy elderly subjects (n=32) with 800 IU/day of dl-α-tocopherol acetate) for 30 days significantly improved delayed-type hypersensitivity (DTH) skin-test response, lymphocyte proliferative response to the T-cell mitogen, as well as T-cell mitogen concanavalin A, and con A- stimulated IL-2 production.[143] In a subsequent study, the same researchers found that supplementation with 400 IU/day of vitamin E for 6 months produced a 91% increase in DTH response of the healthy elderly, which led to the conclusion that this daily dosage is as effective over a more-prolonged period.[144]

During prolonged exercise, vitamin E has been shown to halt the destructive actions of the oxygen-derived free radicals in the cell membranes.[145–148]This was confirmed by the findings of a double-blind, placebo-controlled study that revealed that 300 mg taken daily for a 4-week period significantly reduced markers of lipid peroxidation following an exhaustive bout of cycling,[146] whereas 25 college-age women who received 400 IU daily for 3 weeks prior to a 30-min workout on a treadmill found a difference of 60% between urinary post-exercise (malondialde-hyde) of these women and a non-supplemented control group.[147]

In attempting to identify possible mechanisms for this exercise-induced response to enhanced dietary intake of vitamin E, stimulation of mononuclear cell production of interleukin-1[148] and vitamin E-mediated inhibition of prostaglandin E_2 have been

suggested. The effect of vitamin E supplementation alone on actual clinical mani-
festations of infection in athletes has, however, not yet been investigated.

6.4.4.4 Combinations of Antioxidant Vitamins

Although supplementation with a variety of antioxidant nutrients should theoretically provide greater protection of tissues against exercise-induced oxidative
stress, existing data on humans are contractictory.

In a placebo-controlled study, 12 marathoners were given a combination of
400 IU/day of α–tocopherol and 200 mg/d of ascorbic acid for 4.5 weeks before
participation in a standard marathon. Evidence of lipid peroxidation did not differ
significantly during the 24 h post-race, but creatine kinase levels were significantly
lower in the supplemented group immediately and 24 h after the race.[150]

Vansankari et al.[151] studied the effect of 4 weeks of antioxidant supplementation
(294 mg vitamin E, 1000 mg vitamin C and 60 mg Ubiquinone) vs. placebo supplementation on exercise-induced lipid peroxidation and antioxidant potential
(TRAP) measured in serum and low-density-lipoprotein (LDL) samples following
two 31-km runs in eight endurance athletes. The antioxidant supplementation
resulted in significantly higher α-tocopherol, LDL TRAP, and serum TRAP, but did
not affect the LDL or serum diene concentration.

In the previously described work on participants in the 1993 88-km Comrades
Ultramarathon, [61] it was found that although infection risk was 37% lower in the
group supplementing with a combination of 18 mg β-carotene, 300 mg vitamin C
and 400 IU α-tocopherol per day than in the placebo-supplemented group, the
combination of water-soluble and fat-soluble antioxidants was not more successful
in attenuating the post-exercise infection risk than vitamin C alone. Although the
relatively lower effect of the combined vitamin C, vitamin E and β-carotene supplementation may be attributed to the slow elevation in plasma vitamin E levels and
the fact that this supplementation was not long enough to allow plasma levels to
reach protective status, variance in training and genetic makeup within and between
the groups studied appeared to have an important bearing on the efficacy of antioxidant nutrient supplementation.

In the only laboratory work conducted to date on the effects of combinations
of antioxidants on markers of exercise-induced suppression of immune function,
Pederson et al. (1999)[152] found that administration of a combination of 500 mg of
vitamin C and 400 mg of vitamin E per day did not result in significant changes
in stress hormonal, cytokine, lymphocyte subpopulations or any evidence of non-
specific immunopotentiation or suppression following 1.5 h of downhill running on
a treadmill at 75% of VO_{2max}.

6.5 CONCLUSION: MANAGEMENT OF THE ATHLETE

Current knowledge and research findings appear to support the enhanced dietary
intakes of vitamins B, C, E, and a variety of carotenoid and flavenoid-rich foodstuffs
to raise daily intakes to above the recommended daily requirement for sedentary

individuals.[17] It is well accepted that this is required to meet the increased metabolic requirements of the greater physical work output of athletically active individuals and as a conservative prophylactic measure of increasing resistance to infection in athletes.

Administration of influenza vaccines to athletes to increase their resistance to a multitude of viruses which may only be partially effective depending on how closely the viruses in the vaccine approximate the virus causing the illness.[48] Although antibiotics are more effective in increasing immunocompetence once an infection is present than increased dosage of protective micronutrients, they are also specific to certain bacteria and this needs to be balanced against the modest contribution which supplementation of vitamins may make in increasing resistance to infection.

Indiscriminate supplementation of single antioxidants is not advocated. This is particularly supported in view of the potential hazards associated with excessive intake of fat-soluble vitamins and the uncertainty surrounding the preliminary evidence of pro-oxidative and pro-inflammatory response resulting from administration of excessive quantities of vitamin C. Before an optimal critical threshold level for the various antioxidants is determined, the intake of a well-balanced diet that can be supplemented with the use of balanced multivitamin preparations containing selective ingredients in specified amounts is recommended.

REFERENCES

1. Nieman, D.C., Exercise, upper respiratory infections, and the immune system, *Med. Sci. Sports Exerc.,* 26, 128,1994.
2. Peters, E.M., Exercise, immunology, and upper respiratory tract infections, *Int. J. Sports Med.,* 18, S69, 1997.
3. Nieman, D.C., Nehlsen-Cannarella, S.L., Markoff, P.A., Balk-Lamberton, H., Yang, H., Chritton, D.B.W., Lee, J.W., and Arabatzis, K., The effects of moderate exercise training on natural killer cells and upper respiratory tract infections, *Int. J. Sports Med.,* 11, 467, 1990.
4. Nieman, D.C., Physical activity, fitness and infection, *Exercise and Health: A Consensus of Current Knowledge,* Bouchard, C., Ed., Human Kinetics Publishers, Champaign, IL, 1993.
5. Baron, R.C., Hatch, M.H., Kleeman, K, and MacCormack, J.N., Aseptic meningitis among members of a high school football team. An outbreak associated with echovirus infection, *JAMA,* 248, 1724, 1982.
6. Midveldt, T. and Midvelt, K., Sport and infection, *Scand. J. Soc. Med. Suppl.,* 29, 241, 1982.
7. Girdwood, R.W.A., Infections associated with sport, *Br. J. Sports Med.,* 22, 117, 1988.
8. Smith, J.W. and Weidermann, M.J., The exercise and immunity paradox: A neuroendocrine/cytokine hypothesis, *Med. Sci. Res.,* 18, 749, 1990.
9. Chandra, R.K. and Kumari, S., Nutrition and immunity. An overview, *J. Nutr.,* 12, 1433S, 1994.
10. Machin, L.L., *The Mount Sinai School of Medicine Complete Book of Vitamins.* St. Martins Press, 1997.
11. McGivery, R.W. and Goldstein, G., *Biochemistry. A Functional Approach,* W.B. Saunders, Philadelphia, 1979.

12. Burke, L.M. and Deakin, V., *Clinical Sports Nutrition*, McGraw-Hill Book Company, Sydney, 1994.
13. Hawley, J.A. Dennis, S.C., and Lindsay, F.H., Nutritional practices of athletes; are they sub-optimal? *J. Sport Sci.,* 13S, 75, 1995.
14. Singh, A., Pelletier, P.A., and Deuster, P.A., Dietary requirements for ultra-endurance exercise, *Sports Med.,* 18, 301, 1994.
15. Barry, A., Cantwell, T., Doherty, F., Folan, J.C., Ingoldsby, M., Kevany, J.P., O'Broin, J.D., O'Connor, H., O'Shea, B., Ryan, B.A., and Vaughan, J., A nutritional study of Irish athletes, *Br. J. Sports Med.,* 5, 99, 1981.
16. Blair, S.N., Ellsworth, N.M., Haskell, W.L., Stern, M.P., Farquhar, J.W., and Wood, P.D., Comparison of the nutrient intakes in middle age men and women runners and controls, *Med. Sci. Sports Exerc.,* 13, 310, 1981.
17. American Dietetic Association. Position of the American Dietetic Association: Nutrition for physical fitness and athletic performance for adults, *J. Am. Diet. Assoc.* 87, 933, 1987.
18. Committee on Dietary Allowances, Food and Nutrition Board, National Research Council. Recommended Dietary Allowances. 10th Edition. Washington, DC : National Academic Press, 1989.
19. Cohen, F.L., Potosnak, R.D., Frank, O., and Baker, H.A., Nutritional and hematologic assessment of elite ballet dancers, *Phys. Sports Med.,* 13, 43, 1985.
20. Benson, J., Gillien, D.M., Bourdet, K., and Loosli, A.R., Inadequate nutrition and chronic calorie restriction in adolescent ballerinas, *Phys. Sports Med.,* 10, 79 , 1985.
21. Loosli, A.R., Benson, J., Gillien, D.M., and Bourdet, K., Nutritional habits and knowledge in competive adolescent female gymnasts, *Phys. Sports Med.,* 8, 118, 1986.
22. Burke, L. and Read, R.D.S., Dietary intakes and food use of groups of Australian male triathletes, *Phys. Sports Med.,* 15, 140, 1987.
23. Nieman, D.C., Butler, J.V., Pollett, I.M., Dietrich, S.J., and Lutz, R.D., Nutrient intake of marathoner runners, *J. Am. Diet. Assoc.,* 89, 1273, 1989.
24. Van Erp-Baart, A.M.J., Saris, W.II.M., Binkhorst, R.A., Vos, J.A., and Elvers, J.W.H., Nationwide survey on the nutritional habits in elite athletes, Part I Energy, carbohydrate, protein and fat intake; Part II Mineral and vitamin intake, *Int. J. Sports Med.,* 10, S3, 1989.
25. Singh, A., Evans, P., Gallagher, K.L., and Deuster, P.A., Dietary intakes and biochemical profiles of nutritional status of ultramarathoners, *Med. Sci. Sports. Ex.,* 25, 28, 1993.
26. Niekamp, R.A., and Baer, J.T., In season adequacy of trained cross-country runners, *Int. J. Sports Nutr.,* 5, 45, 1995.
27. Peters, E.M. and Goetzsche, J.M., Dietary practices of South African ultradistance athletes, *Int. J. Sports Nutr.,* 7, 80, 1997.
28. Govender, D., The dietary habits of white and Indian marathon runners in Kwazulu-Natal, RSA. Unpublished master's thesis, 1998.
29. Barnett, D.W. and Conlee, R.K., The effects of commercial dietary supplementation on human performance, *Am. J. Clin. Nutr.,* 40, 586, 1985.
30. Bruce, A., Ekblom, B., and Nilsson, I., The effect of vitamin and mineral supplements in health foods on physical endurance and performance, *Proc. Br. Nutr. Soc.,* 44, 283, 1985.
31. Heath, G.W., Macera, C.A., and Nieman, D.C., Exercise and upper respiratory tract infection: Is there a relationship? *Sports Med.,* 14, 353, 1992.
32. Nieman, D.C., Personal Communication, 1999.

33. Heath, G.W., Ford, E.S., Craven, T.E., Macera, C.A., Jackson, K.L., and Pate, R.R., Exercise and the incidence of upper respiratory tract infections, *Med. Sci. Sports Exerc.*, 23, 152, 1991.
34. Badger, G.F., Dingle, J.H., Feller, A.E., Hodges, R.G., Jordan, W.S., and Rammelkamp, C.H., A study of illness in a group of Cleveland families, *Am. J. Hyg.*, 58, 41, 1953.
35. Fox, J.P., Hall, C.E., Cooney, M.K., Luce, R.E., and Kronmal, R.A., The Seattle virus watch II. Objectives, study population and its observation, data processing and summary of illnesses, *Am. J. Epidemiol.*, 96, 270, 1972.
36. Gwaltney, J.M., Rhinovirus colds: epidemiology, clinical characteristics and transmission, *Eur. J. Respir. Dis.*, 64, 336, 1983.
37. Gwaltney, J.M., Hendley, J.O., Simon, G., and Jordan, W.S., Rhinovirus Infections in an industrial population. I. The occurrence of illness, *N. Engl. J. Med.*, 275, 1262, 1966.
38. Hanson, P.G. and Flaherty, D.K., Immunological responses to training in conditioned runners, *Clin. Sci.*, 60, 215, 1981.
39. Douglas, D.J. and Hanson, P.G., Upper respiratory infections in the conditioned athlete, *Med. Sci. Sports Exerc.*, 10, 55, 1978.
40. Osterback, L. and Qvarnberg, Y., A prospective study of respiratory infections in 12-year-old children actively engaged in sports, *Acta. Physiol. Scand.*, 76, 944, 1987.
41. Schouten, W.J., Vershuur, R., and Kemper, H.C.G., Physical activity and upper respiratory tract infections in a normal population of young men and women. The Amsterdam Growth and Health Study. *Int. J. Sport Med.*, 9, 451, 1988.
42. Nehlsen-Cannarella, S.L., Nieman, D.C., Balk-Lamberton, A.J., Markoff, P.A., Chritton, D.B.Gusewitch, G., and Lee, J.W. The effects of moderate exercise training on immune response, *Med. Sci. Sports Exerc.*, 23, 64, 1991.
43. Nieman, D.C., Miller, A.R., Henson, D.A., Warren, B.J., Gusewitch, G., Johnson, R.L., Davis, J.M., Butterworth, D.E., Herring, J.L., and Nehlsen-Cannarella, S.L., Effect of high- versus moderate-intensity exercise on lymphocyte subpopulations and proliferative response, *Int. J. Sports Med.*, 15, 199, 1994.
44. Nieman, D.C., Nehlsen-Cannarella, S.L., Donohue, K.M., Chritton, D.B., Haddock, B.L., Stout, R.W., and Lee, J.W., The effects of acute moderate exercise on leukocyte and lymphocyte subpopulations, *Med. Sci. Sports Exerc.*, 23, 578, 1991.
45. Nieman, D.C., Tan, S.A., Lee, J.W., and Berk, L.S., Complement and immunoglobin levels in athletes and sedentary controls, *Int. J. Sport. Med.*, 10, 124, 1989.
46. Nieman, D.C., Henson, D.A., Gusewitch, G., Warren, B.J., Dotson, R.C., Butterworth, D.E., and Nehlsen-Cannarella, S.A., Physical activity and immune function in elderly women, *Med. Sci. Sports Exerc.*, 25, 823, 1993.
47. Green, R.L., Kaplan, S.S., Rabin, B.S., Stanitski, C.L., and Zdziarski, U., Immune function in marathon runners, *Ann. Allergy*, 47, 73, 1981.
48. Heiss, F., *Unfallverhutung beim sport*. Shorndorf, K Hoffman, 1971, pp 17–19.
49. Fitsgerald, L., Overtraining increases the susceptibility to infection, *Int. J. Sports Med.*, 12, 369, 1989.
50. Ryan, A.J., Darymple, W., Dull, B.H., Kaden, W.S., and Lerman, S.J., Round table, upper respiratory tract infections in sports, *Phys. Sports Med.*, 3, 29, 1975.
51. Berglund, B. and Hemmingson, P., Infectious disease in elite cross-country skiers; a one-year incidence study, *Clin. Sports Med.*, 2, 19, 1990.
52. Peters, E.M. and Bateman, E.D., Ultramarathon running and upper respiratory tract infections, *S. Afr. Med. J.*, 64, 582, 1983.

53. Peters, E.M., Altitude fails to increase susceptibility of ultramarathon runners to upper respiratory tract infections, *S. Afr. J. Sports Med.*, 5, 4, 1990.
54. Nieman, D.C., Johansen, L.M., Lee, J.W., and Arabatzis, K., Infectious episodes in runners before and after the Los Angeles Marathon, *J. Sports Med. Phys. Fitness,* 30, 316, 1990.
55. Linde, F., Running and upper respiratory tract infections. *Scand. J. Sport Sc.,* 9, 20, 1987.
56. Nash, M.S., Exercise and immunology, *Med. Sci. Sports Exerc.,* 26, 125, 1994.
57. Fitsgerald, L., Exercise and the immune system, *Immunol. Today,* 9, 337, 1988.
58. Nieman, D.C., Johansen, L.M., and Lee, J.W., Infectious episodes in runners before and after a road race, *J. Sports Med. Phys. Fitness,* 29, 289, 1989.
59. Peters, E.M., Campbell, A., and Pawley, L., Vitamin A fails to increase resistance to upper respiratory infection in distance runners, *S. Afr. J. Sports Med.,* 7, 3, 1992.
60. Peters, E.M., Goetzsche, J.M., Grobbelaar, B., and Noakes, T.D., Vitamin C supplementation reduces the incidence of post-race symptoms of upper respiratory tract infection in ultradistance runners, *Am. J. Clin. Nutr.,* 57, 170, 1993.
61. Peters, E.M., Goetzsche, J.M., Joseph, L.E., and Noakes, T.D., Vitamin C as effective as combinations of antioxidant nutrients in reducing symptoms of upper respiratory tract infections in ultramarathon runners, *S. Afr. J. Sports Med.,* 4, 16, 1996.
62. Pyne, D.B., Baker, M.S., Fricker, P.A., McDonald, W.A., Telford, R.D., and Weideman, M.J., Effects of an intensive 12-wk training program by elite swimmers on neutrophil oxidative activity, *Med. Sci. Sports Exerc.,* 27, 536, 1995.
63. Pyne, D.B. and Gleeson, M., Effects of intensive exercise training on immunity in athletes, *Int. J. Sports Med.,* 19, S183, 1998.
64. MacKinnon, L.T., and Hooper, S., Mucosal (secretory) immune system responses to exercise of varying intensity and during overtraining, *Int. J. Sports Med.,* 15, S179, 1994.
65. Gleeson, M., McDonald, W.A., Cripps, A.W., Pyne, D.B., Clancy, R.L., and Fricker, P.A., Exercise, stress, and mucosal immunity of long term intensive training in elite swimmers, *Clin. Exp. Immunol.*, 102, 210, 1995.
66. Nieman, D.C., Exercise, infection and immunity, *Int. J. Sports Med.,* 15, S131, 1995.
67. MacArthy, D.A. and Dale, M.M., The leucocytosis of exercise, *Sports Med.,* 6, 333, 1988.
68. MacKinnon, L.T., *Exercise and Immunology*, Human Kinetics Books, Champaign, IL, 1992.
69. Keast, D., Cameron, K., and Morton, A.R., Exercise and the immune response, *Sports Med.*, 5, 248, 1988.
70. Pederson, B.K., Rohde, T., and Ostowski, K., Recovery of the immune system after exercise, *Acta. Physiol. Scand.*, 162, 325, 1998.
71. Gabriel, H., and Kindermann, W., The acute immune response to exercise; what does it mean? *Int. J. Sports Med.,* 18, S28,1997.
72. Weight, L., Alexander, D., and Jacobs, P., Strenous exercise: analogous to the acute phase response? *Clin. Sci.*, 81, 677, 1991.
73. Cannon, J.G. and Kluger, M.J., Endogenous pyrogen activity in human plasma after exercise, *Science,* 210, 617, 1983.
74. Pyne, D.B., Baker, M.S., Telford, R.D., and Weideman, M, Neutrophil oxidative activity is differentially affected by moderate and intense interval exercise, *Med. Sci. Sports Exerc.* 25 (Suppl), S112, 536, 1995.
75. Pedersen, B.K. and Ullum, H., N K response to physical activity: possible mechanisms of action, *Med. Sci. Sports Exerc.,* 26, 140, 1994.

76. Smith, J.W. and Weidermann, M.J., The exercise and immunity paradox: A neuroendocrine/cytokine hypothesis, *Med. Sci. Res.*, 18, 749, 1990.

77. Shephard, R.J. and Shek, P.N., Impact of physical activity and sport on the immune system, *Rev. Environ. Health*, 11, 133, 1996.

78. Pederson, B.K., Tvede, N., Klarlund, K., Christensen, L.D., Hanse, F.R., Galbo, H., Kharazmi, A., and Halkjer-Kristenen, J., Indomethacin *in vitro* and *in vivo* abolishes post-exercise suppression of natural killer cell activity in peripheral blood, *Int. J. Sports Med.*, 11, 127, 1990.

79. Schwellnus, M., Kiesig, M., Derman., W., and Noakes, T.D., Fusafungine reduces symptoms of upper respiratory tract in infection in runners after a 56 km race, *Med. Sci. Sports Exer.*, 29, S296, 1997.

80. Bendich, A., Vitamins and immunity, *J. Nutr.*, 122, 601, 1992.

81. Anderson, R. and Van Antwerpen, V.L. Vitamins in the maintenance of optimum functions and prevention of phagocyte-mediated tissue damage and carcinogenisis, *Biblio. Nutr. Dieta.*, 52, 66, 1995.

82. Anderson, R., Mechanisms of vitamin-mediated anti-inflammatry and immunomodulatory activity, *Biblio. Nutr. Dieta.*, in press, 1999.

83. Scrimshaw, N.S., Taylor, C.E., and Gordon, J.E., Interaction of nutrition and infection. WHO monograph series no. 57. Geneva. World Health Organization, 1968

84. Green, H.N. and Medllanby, E., Vitamin A as an anti-infective agent, *BJM*, 2, 691, 1928.

85. Bloem, M.W., Wedel, M., Egger, R.J., Speek, A.J., Schrijer, J., Saowakonthha, S., and Scheurs, W., Mild vitamin A deficiency and risk of upper respiratory tract disease and diarrhoea in pre-school and school children in northeastern Thailand, *Am. J. Epidemiol.*, 131, 332, 1990.

86. Hussey, G.D. and Klein, M., A randomized, controlled trial of vitamin A in children with severe measles, *N. Eng. J. Med.*, 323, 160, 1990.

87. Coutsoudis, A., Kiepiela, P., Coovadia, H.M., and Broughton, M., Vitamin A supplementation enhances specific IGA antibody levels and total lymphocyte numbers while improving morbidity in measles, *Paed. Infect. Dis. J.*, 11, 203, 1992.

88. Cramer, W., Drew, A .H., and Mottram, J.C., On the function of the lymphocyte and lymphoid tissue in nutrition, *Lancet* II, 1202, 1921.

89. Rall, L.C. and Meydani, S.N., Vitamin B_6 and immune competence, *Nutr. Rev.*, 51, 217, 1993.

90. Miller, L.T. and Kerkvliet, N.L., Effect of vitamin B_6 on immunocompetence in the elderly, *Ann. N.Y. Acad. Sci.*, 587, 49, 1990.

91. Meydani, S.N., Ribaya-Mercado, J.D., Russel, R.M., Sahyoun, N., Morrow, F.D., and Gershoff, S.N., Vitmin B_6 deficiency impairs interleukin -2 production and lymphocyte proliferation in elderly adults, *Am. J. Clin. Nutr.*, 53, 1275, 1991.

92. Rokitzki, L., Sagredos, A.N., Resuss, F., Buchner, M., and Keul, J., Acute changes in vitamin B_6 status in endurance athletes before and after a marathon, *Int. J. Sports Nutr.*, 4, 154, 1994.

93. Rook, G.W., The role of vitamin D in tuberculosis, *Am. Rev. Resp. Dis.*, 138, 768, 1988.

94. Young, M.R.I., Haplin, J., Wang, J., Wright, M.A., Mathews, J., and Pak, A.S., 1α, 25-dihydroxyvitamin D3 plus γ-interferon blocks lung tumor production of granulocyte-macrophage colony-stimulating factor and induction of immunosuppressor cells, *Cancer Res.*, 53, 6006, 1993.

95. Alessio, H.M., Exercise-induced oxidative stress, *Med. Sci. Sports Exerc.*, 25, 208, 1993.

96. Peters, E.M., Antioxidant nutrient supplementation and prolonged exercise, *The Leech*, 62, 1993.
97. Peters, E.M., Exercise induced toxicity ... is antioxidant supplementation the answer? *Micronutrients*, May, 1996.
98. Anderson, R.D., Phagocyte-derived oxidants as mediators of inflammation-associated damage, *S. Afr. J. Sci.*, 87, 594, 1991.
99. Peters, E.M., Vitamin C, neutrophil function and upper respiratory tract infection risk in distance runners. The missing link, *Ex. Immunol. Rev.*, 3, 32, 1997.
100. Mars, M., Govender, S., Weston, A., Naidoo, V., and Chuturgoon, A., High intensity exercise: a cause of lymphocyte apoptosis? *Biochem. Biophys. Res. Com.*, 249, 366,1998
101. Goldfarb, A.G., Antioxidants: role of supplementation to prevent exercise-induced oxidative stress, *Med. Sci. Sports Exerc.*, 25, 232, 1992.
102. Murata, T., Tamai, H., and Morinobo, T., Determination of β-carotene in plasma, blood cells and buccal mucosa by electrochemical detection, *Lipids*, 27, 840, 1992.
103. Gilbert, A.M., Stitch, H.F., Rosin, M.P., and Davidson, A.J. Variation in the uptake of beta carotene in the oral mucosa of individuals after 3 days of supplementation, *Int. J. Cancer*, 45, 855, 1990.
104. Boosalis, M.G., Snowdon, D.A., Tully, C.L., and Gross, M.D., Acute phase response and plasma carotenoid concentrations in older women: findings from the Nun study, *Nutr.*, 1212, 475, 1996.
105. Sies, H. and Stahl, W., Vitamins E and C, β–carotene, and other carotenoids as antioxidants, *Am. J. Clin. Nutr.*, 62,1315S, 1995.
106. Fotouhi, N., Meydani, M., Santos, M.S., Meydani, S.M., Hennekens, C.H., Gaziano, J.M, Carotenoid and tocopherol concentrations in plasma, peripheral blood polynuclear mononuclear cells, and red blood cells after long-term β-carotene supplementation in men, *Am. J. Clin. Nutr.*, 63, 553,1996.
107. Moolla, M.E., The effect of supplemental antioxidants on the incidence and severity of upper respiratory tract infections in ultramarathoners, Unpublished master's thesis, University of Cape Town, 1996.
108. Bendich, A., Carotenoids and Immunity, *Clin. Appl. Nutr.*, 1, 45, 1991.
109. Frei, B., England, L., and Ames, B.N., Ascorbate is an outstanding antioxidant in human blood plasma, *Proc. Nation. Acad. Sci.*, 86, 6377, 1989.
110. Evans, R., Currie, L., and Campbell, A., The distribution of ascorbic acid between various cellular components of blood in normal individuals, and its relation to the plasma concentration, *Br. J. Nutr.*, 47, 473, 1982.
111. Anderson, R., Effects of ascorbate on normal and abnormal leukocyte functions, *Vitamin C. New Clinical Applications in Immunology, Lipid Metabolism and Cancer*, Hanck, A., Bern Hans Huber, 1982, 23.
112. Anderson, R. and Lukey, P.T., A biological role for ascorbate in the selective neutralization of extracellular, phagocyte derived reactive oxidants, *Ann. N.Y. Acad. Sci*, 498, 219, 1987.
113. Heraczynska-Cedro, K., Wartanowicz, M., Panczenko-Kresowska, B., Cedro, K., Klosiewicz-Wasek, B., and Wasek, W., Inhibitory effect of vitamins C and E on the free radical production in human polymorphonuclear leukocytes, *Eur. J. Clin. Invest.*, 24, 316, 1994.
114. Chretien, J.H. and Garagusi, V.F., Correction of corticosteroid-induced defects of polymorphonuclear neutrophil function by ascorbic acid, *J. Reticulo. Soc.*, 14, 280, 1973.

115. Jariwalla, R.J. and Harakeh, S., Antiviral and immunomodulatory activities of ascorbic acid, *Subcell. Biochem.*, 25, 17, 1996.
116. Hemila, H., Vitamin C and the common cold, *Br. J. Nutr.*, 65, 3, 1992.
117. Pauling, L., The significance of the evidence about ascorbic acid and the common cold, *Proc. Nat. Acad. Sci.*, 68, 2678, 1971
118. Hemila, H., Vitamin C and Infectious Diseases, *Vitamin C. The State of the Art in Disease Prevention Sixty Years After the Nobel Prize*, Poaletti, R., Sies, H., Bug, J., Grossi, E., Poli, A., Springer-Verlag , Milano, 1998, 74.
119. Hemila, H., Does vitamin C alleviate the symptoms of the common cold? A review of the current evidence, *Scand. J. Infec. Dis.*, 26, 1, 1994.
120. Hemila H., Vitamin C supplementation and common cold symptoms: problems with inaccurate reviews, *Nutr.*, 12, 804, 1996.
121. Hemila, H., Vitamin C intake and susceptibility to the common cold, *J. Nutr.*, 77, 59, 1997.
122. Hemila H., Vitamin C and common cold incidence: a review of studies with subjects under heavy stress, *Int. J. Sports Med.*, 17, 379, 1996.
123. Bessel-Lorck, C., Common cold prophylaxis in young people at a ski camp (in German), *Medizinische,* 44, 2126, 1959.
124. Kimbarowski, J.A. and Mokrow, N.J., Coloured precipitation reaction of the urine according to Kimbarowski (FARK) as an index of the effect of ascorbic acid during treatment of viral influenza (in German), *Dtsch. Gesundheitssw,* 22, 2413, 1967.
125. Ritzel, G., Critical analysis of the role of vitamin C in the prophylaxis and treatment of the common cold (in German), *Helvetica Medica Acta,* 28, 63, 1961.
126. Ritzel, G., Ascorbic acid and the common cold (letter), *JAMA*, 235, 1108, 1976.
127. Sabiston, B.H. and Radomski, M.W., Health problems and vitamin C in Canadian Northern Military Operations. DCIEM Report NO 74-R-1012. Downsview, Ontario, Defense Research Board, 1974. *Int. J. Sports Med.*, 17, 379, 1996.
128. Hunt, C., Chakaravorty, N.K., Annan, G., Habibzadeh, N., and Schorah, C.J., The clinical effects of vitamin C supplementation in elderly hospitalized with acute respiratory infections, *Int. J. Vit. Nutr. Res.,* 64, 202, 1994.
129. Pitt, H.A. and Costrini, A.M., Vitamin C prophylaxis in marine recruits, *JAMA,* 241, 908, 1979.
130. Nieman, D.C., Henson, D.A., Butterworth, D.E., Warren, B.J., Davis, J.M., Fagoaga, O.R., and Nehlsen-Cannarella, S.L., Vitamin C supplementation does not alter the immune response to 2.5 hours of running, *Int. J. Sports Nutr.,* 7, 173, 1997.
131. Alessio, H.M., Goldfarb, A.H., and Cao, G., Exercise-induced oxidative stress before and after vitamin C supplementation, *Int. J. Sports Nutr.*, 7, 1, 1997.
132. Peters, E.M. and Anderson, R., Apparent enhancement of exercise induced acute-phase protein response following vitamin C supplementation in athletes participating in an 88-km event, *Int. J. Sports Med.,* in press.
133. Herbert, V., Viewpoint. Does mega-C do more good than harm, or more harm than good? *Nutr. Today,* Jan/Feb, 29, 1993.
134. Salonen, J.T., Nyyssonen, K., Korpela, H., Tuomilehto, J., Seppanen, R., and Salonen, R., High stored iron levels are associated with excess risk of myocardial infarction in Eastern Finnish men, *Circulation*, 2, 803, 1992.
135. Shilotri, P.G. and Bhat, K.S., The effect of mega doses of vitamin C on bacteriocidal activity of leukocytes, *Am. J. Clin. Nutr.*, 30, 1077, 1977.
136. Podmore, I.D., Griffiths, H.R., Herbert, K.E., Mistry, N., Mistry, P., and Lunec, J., Pro-oxidant effect of vitamin C, *Nature,* 6676, 559, 1998.

137. Levine, M., Duruvala, C., Park, J.P., Rumsey, S.C., and Wang, Y., Does vitamin C have a pro-oxidant effect? *Nature*, 6676, 559, 1998.
138. Anderson, R., Smit, M.J., Joone G.K., and Van Staden A.M. Vitamin C and cellular immune functions. *Ann. NY Acad. Sci., 587, 34, 1990.*
139. Orr, C.W.M., Studies on ascorbic acid. 1. Factors influencing ascorbate mediated inhibition of catalase. *Biochem.*, 6, 2995, 1967.
140. Poulsen, H.E., Weiman, A., Salonen, K.N., Loft, S., Cadet, J., Douki, T., and Ravanat, J.L., Does vitamin C have a pro-oxidant effect? *Nature*, 6676, 559, 1998.
141. Meydani, M., Evans, W.J., Handelman, G., Biddle, L., Fielding, R.A., Meydani, S.N., Burrill, J., Fiatarone, M.A., Blumberg, J.B., and Cannon, J.G., Protective effect of vitamin E on exercise-induced oxidative damage in young and older adults, *Am. J. Physiol.*, 264, R992, 1993.
142. Latshaw, J.D., Nutrition-mechanisns of immunosuppression, *Vet. Immunopathol.* 30, 111, 1991.
143. Meydani, S.N., Barklund P.M., Liu S., Vitamin E supplementation enhances cell mediated immunity in elderly subjects, *Am. J. Clin. Nutr.,* 52, 557, 1990.
144. Meydani, M., Meydani, S.N., Leka, L., Gong, J., and Blumberg, J.B., Effect of long term vitamin E supplementation on lipid peroxidation and immune responses of young and old subjects, *FASEB J*, 67, A415, 1993.
145. Packer, L., Vitamin E, physical exercise and tissue damage in animals, *Med. Biol.,* 62, 105, 1984.
146. Sudmilla, S.K., Tanaka, H., Kitao, H., and Nakadoma, F., Exercise-induced lipid peroxidation and leakage of enzymes before and after vitamin E supplementation, *Int. J. Biochem.*, 21, 835, 1989.
147. Jenkins, R.R.R., Proceedings of the panel discussion: antioxidants and the elite athlete, Dallas, Texas, 1992.
148. Cannon, J.G., Meydani, S.N., Fielding ,R.A., Fiatarone, M.A., Meydani, M., Farhang-mehr, M., Orencole, S.F., Blumberg, J.B., Evans, W.J., Acute phase response in exercise II. Association between vitamin E, cytokines, and muscle proteolysis. *Am. J. Physiol.*, 260, R1235, 1991.
149. Prasad, J.S., Effect of vitamin E supplementation on leukocyte function. *Am. J. Clin. Nutr., 33, 606, 1980.*
150. Rokitzki, L., Logeman, E., Sagredos, A.N., Murphy, M., Wetzel-Roth, W., and Keul, J., Lipid peroxidation and antioxidant vitamins under extreme endurance stress, *Acta. Physiol. Scand.* 151, 149, 1994.
151. Vasankari, T.J., Kujala, U.M., Vasakari, T.M., Vuorimaa, T., and Ahotupa, M., Increased serum and low density-lipoprotein antioxidant potential after antioxidant supplementation in endurance athletes, *Am. J. Clin. Nutr.*, 65, 1052,1997.
152. Pederson, B.K., Personal communication, 1999.

CHAPTER 7

Minerals and Exercise Immunology

Michael Gleeson

CONTENTS

7.1 INTRODUCTION

A mineral is an inorganic element, usually solid, found in nature. In nutrition, the term mineral is usually used to classify those dietary elements essential to life processes. Inadequate mineral nutrition has been associated with a variety of human diseases including anemia, cancer, diabetes, hypertension, osteoporosis and tooth decay.[1-5] Thus, appropriate dietary intake of essential minerals is necessary for optimal health and physical performance.

Some minerals have an essential role in the functioning of immune cells. Minerals are classified as macrominerals or microminerals (trace elements) based on the extent of their occurrence in the body and the amounts needed in the diet. Macrominerals (e.g., sodium, calcium, magnesium, phosphorus) each constitute at least

1-8493-0741-4/00/$0.00+$.50
© 2000 by CRC Press LLC

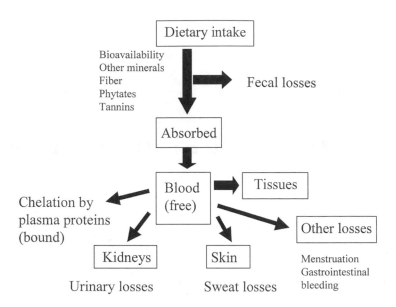

Figure 7.1 Factors affecting absorption and tissue distribution of minerals. Note that exercise may increase losses of minerals in urine and sweat and that several other components of the diet may interfere with mineral absorption.

0.01% of total body mass. The trace elements each compose less than 0.001% of total body mass and are needed in quantities of less than 100 mg per day. Fourteen trace elements have been identified as essential for maintenance of health and several are known to exert modulating effects on immune function, including iron, zinc, copper, and selenium (Table 7.1). Deficiencies of one or more of these trace elements are associated with immune dysfunction and increased incidence of infection.[1,6–10]

A temporary depression of the free (unbound) plasma concentration of some trace elements (e.g. iron, zinc, copper) may occur following prolonged exercise due to redistribution to other tissue compartments (e.g. erythrocytes and leukocytes), or to the release of chelating proteins from granulocytes or the liver as part of the acute-phase response (Figure 7.1). Regular exercise, particularly in a hot environment, incurs increased losses of some of these minerals in sweat and urine,[11–13] which means that the daily requirement is increased in athletes engaged in heavy training.[11–15] However, with the exception of iron and zinc, isolated deficiencies of minerals are rare. Iron deficiency is reported to be the most widespread micronutrient deficiency in the world,[8,9] and field studies consistently associate iron deficiency with increased morbidity from infectious disease.[2,8,9,16] Furthermore, exercise has a pronounced effect on both iron and zinc metabolism. As such, the present discussion will focus mainly on these two trace elements, although the impact of exercise on other minerals known to be important for immune function–including magnesium, copper and selenium–will also be considered.

Table 7.1   Minerals with Established Roles in Immune Function and Effects of Dietary Deficiency or Excess

Mineral	Role in immune function	Effect of deficiency	Effect of excess
Copper	Normal iron absorption Co-factor of Superoxide dismutase(antioxidant)	Anemia Impaired immune function	Nausea, vomiting
Iron	Oxygen transport Metalloenzymes	Anemia Increased infections	Hemochromatosis, liver cirrhosis, heart disease, more infections
Magnesium	Protein synthesis Metalloenzymes	Muscle weakness, fatigue, apathy, muscle tremor and cramp	Nausea, vomiting, diarrhea
Selenium	Co-factor of Glutathione Peroxidase (antioxidant)	Cardiomyopathy, cancer, heart disease, impaired immune function, erythrocyte fragility	Nausea, vomiting, fatigue, hair loss
Zinc	Metalloenzymes, protein synthesis, antioxidant	Impaired growth and healing, increased infections, anorexia	Impaired absorption of Fe and Cu, increased HDL-C/LDL-C ratio, anemia, nausea, vomiting, immune system impairment

7.2 IRON

The RDA for iron is 10 mg for males and 15 mg for females. Major dietary sources of iron are shown in Table 7.2. Iron deficiency is prevalent throughout the world and by some estimates, as much as 25% of the world's population is iron deficient.[8] Within the athletic population, studies show that it is male and female endurance athletes who may be iron depleted.[17-20] Endurance competitors risk potential iron deficiency because of the involvement of transferrin (the iron-transporting polypeptide found in plasma) in antioxidant reactions and additional iron losses in sweat, urine and feces. However, the proportion of athletes who are iron depleted is no greater than in the general (mostly sedentary) population,[19] implying that part of the reason for low iron status in athletes may be unrelated to exercise—for example, poor diet or loss of iron during menstruation, although many elite female endurance athletes are amenorrheic.

Nevertheless, exercise may contribute to an iron-depleted state; the acute-phase host response to stress (including exercise) involves the depression of circulating free iron levels.[8] This exercise-induced fall in plasma-free iron has been reported by

Table 7.2 Dietary Sources and Daily Recommended Dietary Allowances (RDA) or Estimated Safe and Adequate Daily Dietary Intake (ESADDI) of Minerals Known to Be Important for Immune Function

Mineral	Source	RDA or ESADDI*	% Absorbed
Iron	Liver, kidney, eggs, red meats, seafood, oysters, bread, flour, molasses, dried legumes, nuts, leafy green vegetables, broccoli, figs, raisins, cocoa	10 mg (males) 15 mg (females)	10–30 (heme iron) 2–10 (non-heme iron)
Zinc	Oysters, shellfish, beef, liver, poultry, dairy products, whole grains, wheat germ, vegetables, asparagus, spinach	15 mg (males) 12 mg (females)	20–50
Magnesium	Seafood, nuts, green leafy vegetables, fruits, Whole grain products, milk, yogurt	420 mg (males) 320 mg (females)	25–60
Copper	Liver, kidney, shellfish, meat, fish, poultry, eggs, bran cereals, nuts, legumes, broccoli, banana, avocado, chocolate	1.5–3.0 mg*	20–50
Selenium	Meat, liver, kidney, poultry, fish, dairy produce, seafood, whole grains and nuts from selenium-rich soil	70 μg (males) 55 μg (females)	?
Manganese	Whole grains, peas and beans, leafy vegetables, bananas	2.0–5.0 mg	?

several authors,[21, 22] although it should be noted that lower values in athletes may be explained, at least in part, by the plasma volume expansion associated with exercise training.[18] The elevation of circulating cytokines including IL-1, IL-6, and TNF-α by inflammation, infection, stress, or prolonged strenuous exercise causes increased uptake and storage of iron into monocytes and macrophages and stimulates release of the iron-binding protein lactoferrin from granulocytes within the circulation.[23–25] Lactoferrin is then thought to chelate iron from transferrin, forming lactoferrin–iron complexes, leading to a depression of plasma-free iron concentration that is independent of plasma volume changes.

Iron, as a component of hemoglobin, myoglobin, and cytochromes, is essential for oxidative metabolism. The immune system itself appears to be particularly sensitive to the availability of iron.[26] Iron deficiency has neither completely harmful nor enhancing effects on immune function. On the one hand, free iron is necessary for bacterial growth—removal of iron with the help of chelating agents such as lactoferrin reduces bacterial multiplication, particularly in the presence of specific antibodies.[5] For example, iron-deficient mice had a lower rate of mortality after infection with *salmonella* than mice who were iron-replete.[16] In view of such findings, iron deficiency may actually protect an individual from infection, whereas supplementation might predispose the individual to infectious disease, particularly because a high intake of iron can impair gastrointestinal zinc absorption. Iron also catalyses the production of hydroxyl free radicals and this may be a cause of the apparently increased risk of chronic diseases such as coronary heart disease in persons with high intakes of iron.[27] There is growing evidence that iron overload is associated with increased risk for several chronic inflammatory diseases. Free radicals may cause damage to cell membranes, proteins, and nucleic acids. Since physical exercise is associated with increased production of reactive oxygen species (ROS), a higher rate of production of free radicals due to excessive iron intake may lead to an augmentation of exercise-induced oxidative stress.[28] Iron overload may also have some effects on T-lymphocyte distribution, which could be interpreted as being detrimental to host defense. In rodents, excessive intakes of iron led to a decreased ratio of T-helper/T-cytotoxic cells in both the spleen and the circulation.[29]

On the other hand, iron deficiency depresses various aspects of immune function including the lymphocyte-proliferative response to mitogens, delayed cutaneous hypersensitivity, macrophage IL-1 production, and natural killer cell cytotoxic activity;[2,5,8,30,31] the latter possibly owing to the reduced production of interferon associated with iron deficiency.[8] Blood neutrophil phagocytic function is impaired by low iron availability, as evidenced by decreased bactericidal killing, lowered myeloperoxidase activity and a decrease in the oxidative burst.[9] In contrast, high concentrations of ferric ions inhibit phagocytosis of human neutrophils *in vitro*.[32, 33] The appropriate conclusion from the studies cited above is that *both* iron deficiency and iron overload may impair immune function.

A number of causes of iron-deficiency in endurance athletes involved in heavy training have been suggested. Exercise may cause reductions in gastrointestinal iron absorption[17] and iron is lost at a rate of about 0.3 mg/l in sweat (Table 7.3);[17] this could contribute to losses of up to 2 mg of iron per day in athletes who are training extensively in a hot environment. To replace iron losses, intakes need to be about 10 times greater than the amounts lost since, on average, only about 10% of ingested dietary iron is absorbed. Thus, it would take about 3 mg of dietary iron to replace the iron lost in one liter of sweat. About 60% of iron in animal tissues is in the heme form–that is iron associated with hemoglobin and myoglobin—and thus is found only in animal foods. Non-heme iron is found in both animal and plant foods. Heme iron is absorbed better than non-heme iron. About 10%–30% of ingested heme iron is absorbed in the gut, whereas only about 2%–10% of non-heme iron gets absorbed (Table 7.3).[34] This example illustrates an important point, i.e., that the bioavailability of many minerals is influenced by the form in which they are consumed. Some substances found in foods may promote or inhibit absorption of minerals (Figure 7.1). For example, Vitamin C prevents the oxidation of ferrous iron (Fe^{2+}) to the ferric (Fe^{3+}) form.[34] Ferrous iron is more readily absorbed, thus facilitating non-heme-iron absorption, but has no effect on the absorption of heme iron. Thus, drinking a glass of fresh orange juice will improve the absorption of iron from bread or cereals. Some natural substances found in foods such as tannins (e.g. in tea), phosphates, phytates, oxalates, and excessive fiber may decrease the bioavailability of non-heme iron.[34]

Another route of increased iron loss in athletes could be through damage to erythrocytes and increased loss of hemoglobin in the urine. Elevations in plasma

Table 7.3   Body Content and Body Fluid Concentrations of Minerals Known to be Important for Immune Function

Mineral	Symbol	Total Amount in Body (mg)	Body fluid concentration (mg/l)		
			Serum	Sweat	Urine
Iron	Fe	5000	0.4–1.4	0.3–0.4	0.1–0.15
Zinc	Zn	2000	0.7–1.3	0.7–1.3	0.2–0.5
Magnesium	Mg	25000	16–30	4–34	60–100
Copper	Cu	100	0.7–1.7	0.2–0.6	0.03–0.04
Selenium	Se	13	0.05– 0.10		
Manganese	Mn	12	<0.02		

ferritin over the first 2 days of a 20-day road race have been attributed to the intravascular hemolysis that occurs with "foot strike" as the increases coincide with falls in hemoglobin levels.[35] This loss of hemoglobin is often evidenced by a slight red coloration of the urine and is also known as "march hemoglobinuria." However, foot-strike hemolysis has also been reported to be a negligible drain on iron stores.[18] Some athletes are also susceptible to gastrointestinal bleeding during exercise, which may increase fecal iron losses. In summary, athletes who are engaged in heavy training are likely to lose 50%–75% more iron in sweat, urine, and feces than sedentary individuals.

The low bioavailability of iron in vegetarian diets possibly also contributes to lower serum ferritin levels in athletes consuming a modified vegetarian diet. Iron may also be short in a lactovegetarian diet because of the absence of heme-iron. However, a number of studies have failed to find that exercise per se decreased iron status,[20, 36] although this may be attributed to the relatively low training volumes employed. The consensus is that all athletes should be aware of heme-iron-rich foods such as lean red meat, poultry, and fish and include them in the daily diet. Distance runners are recommended to have daily iron intakes of 17.5 mg/day for men and around 23 mg/day for normally menstruating women,[19] assuming iron absorption to be 10% of dietary iron presented. These requirements can be met through consumption of a well-balanced diet sufficient to meet daily energy requirements. Studies on different groups of athletes[37, 38] have shown that iron intake is proportional to energy intake (Figure 7.2), such that athletes consuming in excess of 10 MJ per day from a varied food base will obtain the RDA for iron. Thus, endurance athletes who match their energy intake (from varied food sources) to their energy expenditure are likely to obtain more than enough iron. Those at risk of poor iron status are those athletes consuming low energy intakes or avoiding food sources rich in heme iron. Vegetarian athletes should ensure that plant-food choices are iron-dense, for example, green leafy vegetables. Breakfast cereals are usually fortified with iron and provide a good source of this mineral.

Megadoses of iron are not advised and routine oral iron supplements should not be taken without medical advice. Only where there is laboratory confirmation of

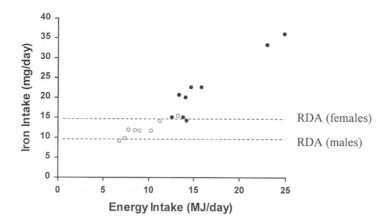

Figure 7.2   The relationship between mean daily intake of dietary energy and iron in male (closed circles) and female (open circles) athletes. Each point represents a mean value for a group. Data from Erp-Baart et al.[37] and Fogelholm.[38]

very low iron status and/or iron-deficient anemia is there a need for iron supplements. Prolonged consumption of large amounts of iron can cause a disturbance in iron metabolism in susceptible individuals with an accumulation of iron in the liver.[39] Hepatic iron accumulates as hemosiderin, which in excess can cause hemochromatosis in the 0.2%–0.3% of the population who are genetically predisposed.[40] This condition causes cirrhosis and can be fatal.[40] Excess intake of iron may also lead to reduced absorption of other divalent cations, particularly zinc and copper.[7, 8, 12] Groups at risk of insufficient iron intake who may be suitable candidates for iron supplementation include female endurance athletes, gymnasts, vegetarians, and those undergoing restricted energy intakes.

7.3   ZINC

The role of zinc in immune function has received increasing attention in recent years. Zinc is essential for the development of the immune system and more than 100 metalloenzymes have been identified as zinc-dependent, including those involved in the transcription of DNA to RNA and the synthesis of proteins.[41] For example, zinc is a co-factor for the enzyme terminal deoxynucleotidyl transferase, which is required by immature T-cells for their replication and functioning. Zinc also plays a key role in the antioxidant defense system as a component of metallothionin and a cofactor of Cu-Zn-superoxide dismutase. Zinc is also required for the optimum activity of some hormones (e.g., growth hormone[42] and thymulin[43]) and the binding of zinc to ligands in membranes seems to be essential for maintaining the structural integrity of their protein and lipid components.[44]

The RDA for zinc is 15 mg for males and 12 mg for females. The major dietary sources of zinc are shown in Table 7.2. The effects of severe zinc deficiency on immune function include lymphoid atrophy, decreased delayed-hypersensitivity cutaneous responses, decreased IL-2 production, impaired mitogen-stimulated lymphocyte proliferative responses and decreased natural killer-cell cytotoxic activity (NKCA).[1, 8, 30] Furthermore, zinc availability affects superoxide free radical production by stimulated macrophages and neutrophils,[45] although in the *in vitro* situation, this effect seems to depend on the actual molecular form of zinc.[46] Even mild zinc deficiency has been associated with impaired immune function in humans. Although the immunological changes were less severe than in the state of chronic malnutrition, the T-helper/T-cytotoxic cell ratio, NKCA, IL-1 and IL-2 production by mononuclear cells and thymulin activity were reduced in humans during mild zinc deficiency.[47] Thymulin, a hormone dependent on zinc for its normal biological activity, is secreted from the thymus gland and is essential for the normal development and proliferation of lymphoid tissue and the maturation of lymphocytes.

Vegetarian athletes are at risk of zinc deficiency because meat and seafoods are rich sources of zinc. Although nuts, legumes, and whole-grain cereals are also good sources of zinc, the high levels of fiber in these foods can decrease zinc absorption.[34] Zinc deficiency could also be a problem for athletes in sports where a low body mass is thought to confer a performance advantage. Very-low-energy or starvation-type diets will obviously restrict zinc intake and in athletes engaged in regular strenuous exercise, zinc losses will also be increased.

Following an acute bout of strenuous exercise, the plasma zinc concentration may increase—possibly as a result of leakage from damaged muscle or, more likely, erythrocytes.[48, 49] Anderson et al[13] found that serum zinc concentration was unchanged immediately after a 6-mile run, but had decreased significantly by 2 h post-exercise. It appears that post-exercise changes in plasma zinc concentration are sensitive to the zinc status of the individual. Lukaski et al[50] have suggested that there is an impairment in the mobilization of zinc from tissues in zinc-depleted persons. Reduced plasma zinc concentrations have been reported following physical and mental stress, infections, and inflammation. Like iron, an acute phase response seems to be associated with reduced plasma levels of zinc, but falls in zinc after exercise may rather reflect a redistribution of zinc to the liver and erythrocytes and increased urinary loss.[51] As zinc is lost from the body mainly in sweat and urine (Table 7.3) and these losses are increased by exercise, it is possible that a heavy schedule of exercise training could induce a zinc deficiency in athletes. Although daily losses may be small in relation to the total body content of zinc, any losses must be replaced by an intake two to five times greater than the losses incurred, as only 20%-50% of ingested dietary zinc is absorbed. Highly trained women excreted more zinc in their urine over a 3-day observation period than untrained controls[35] and an acute 60-minute bout of intermittent high-intensity exercise increased 24-hour urinary zinc excretion by 34% compared with a resting day in well trained male games players.[52] Moreover, male and female athletes tend to have lower plasma zinc concentrations than untrained subjects: in one study 29% of female runners had mean plasma zinc concentrations below the normal range (0.7–1.3 mg/l).[49]

Athletes' diets typically contain less zinc per kilojoule ingested, with female athletes appearing to have lower zinc intakes than their male counterparts.[53, 54] Diets rich in refined carbohydrate are usually somewhat deficient in zinc.[41] In addition, exercise-induced alterations in gastrointestinal function may restrict zinc absorption,

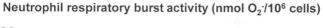

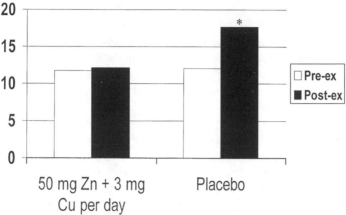

Figure 7.3   The effect of zinc and copper supplementation vs. placebo on the exercise-induced change in neutrophil respiratory burst activity. Data from Singh et al.[41]

as may a diet high in iron intake (>40 mg/day).[55] This is an example of one of the potential problems associated with taking isolated mineral supplements: An increased intake of one mineral may interfere with the absorption of another. However, it should be realized that experiments using serum or plasma zinc levels alone to assess zinc nutritional status are subject to limitations as this level can be influenced by a number of factors other than dietary zinc intake, including the time since the last meal, gender, diurnal variations, pregnancy, use of oral contraceptives, use of corticosteriods, infection, and exercise.[54–57] A better index of zinc status is provided by measurement of erythrocyte zinc concentration, which is about 10 times that found in the plasma.[51]

It is possible that some of the immune function changes seen after prolonged strenuous exercise are related to zinc deficiency or to an exercise-induced transient fall in plasma zinc concentration.

However, studies concerning the relationship between immune function, exercise and zinc status in athletes are lacking. Certainly, more research is needed in this area. However, a recent study in male runners found that 6 days of zinc supplementation (25 mg zinc and 1.5 mg copper twice a day) had a dual effect: Supplementation inhibited the exercise-associated increase in superoxide free radical formation by activated neutrophils (Figure 7.3) and exaggerated the exercise-induced suppression of T-lymphocyte proliferation in response to phytohaemagglutinin or concanavalin-A.[41] The authors interpreted this to mean that zinc both potentiates and protects against exercise-induced immunosuppression; on the one hand, zinc supplements exaggerate exercise-induced suppression of the T-lymphocyte proliferative response, perhaps temporarily predisposing the individual to opportunistic infection, and on the other, zinc supplements protect the individual against the harmful effects of ROS. However, if zinc supplementation inhibits ROS release from activated neutrophils and monocytes, this could also be interpreted as meaning that the killing power of these cells is impaired, thus also rendering the individual more susceptible to infection. Recent reports suggest that zinc supplementation in humans increases resistance to upper respiratory tract infection.[58]

Megadoses of zinc have further detrimental effects on immune function. The administration of zinc (150 mg twice a day) to 11 healthy males for a 6-week period was associated with reduced T-lymphocyte proliferative responses to mitogen stimulation and impaired polymorphonuclear cell phagocytic and chemotaxic activity.[59] In contrast, zinc in much higher than normal physiological concentrations (20 mg/l, compared with ~1 mg/l in extracellular fluids) did not affect human neutrophil phagocytic activity *in vitro*.[60]

High doses of zinc (>25 mg per day) impair the absorption of other essential minerals, including iron and copper.[34] In view of the evidence from human studies carried out *in vivo,* megadoses of zinc are not recommended. Athletes should be encouraged to include zinc-rich foods in the diet, e.g., poultry, meat, fish, and dairy products. On the basis of available evidence, zinc supplementation is not warranted for most athletes. Vegetarians have been recommended to take a 10–20 mg supplement of zinc daily but in view of the findings of Singh et al.[41] supplements at the lower end of this range may be more suitable for vegetarian athletes. As a general rule, if supplements are to be taken by athletes, they should not exceed the RDA for any mineral.

7.4 OTHER MINERALS

7.4.1 Magnesium

Magnesium, an essential cofactor for many enzymes involved in biosynthetic processes and energy metabolism, is required for normal neuromuscular coordination.[61–63] The total body content of magnesium is about 25 g (Table7.3). The RDA for magnesium is 420 mg/day for men and 320 mg/day for women, hence, magnesium is classified as a macromineral rather than a trace element. The main dietary sources of magnesium are listed in Table 7.2. Most studies of dietary habits in athletes suggest that magnesium intake exceeds the RDA.[12] However, it should always be borne in mind that the data used to determine RDAs for micronutrients often did not include athletes, or the activity levels of the subjects were not reported. Therefore, while the RDAs may apply to the sedentary population, they may not be an accurate means of evaluating the nutritional needs of individuals engaged in regular strenuous exercise. Several studies have reported low serum magnesium concentrations in athletes[64, 65] and it is clear that prolonged strenuous exercise is associated with increased losses of magnesium in urine and sweat.[66] Although, as with zinc and iron, it is extremely unlikely that a single bout of exercise will induce substantial magnesium losses, it is possible that a state of mild magnesium deficiency could be induced during a period of heavy training, particularly in a warm environment where sweat losses will be high.

Magnesium deficiency in both humans and animals is associated with neuromuscular abnormalities including muscle weakness, cramps and structural damage of muscle fibers and organelles.[63, 67] This may be due to an impairment of calcium homeostasis secondary to an oxygen free-radical-induced alteration in the integrity of the membrane of the sarcoplasmic reticulum.[68] A lack of magnesium may also be associated with a depletion of selenium and reduced glutathione peroxidase activity, which would be expected to increase the susceptibility to damage by free radicals.[69] Hence, it is possible that magnesium deficiency may potentiate exercise-induced muscle damage and stress responses, but direct evidence for this is lacking. Magnesium deficiency exacerbates the inflammatory state following ischemic insult to the myocardium and it has been suggested that this is due to a substance-P-mediated increase in the secretion of proinflammatory cytokines in the magnesium-deficient state.[70, 71] It has yet to be determined if magnesium status affects the cytokine response to exercise in humans.

7.4.2 Copper and Selenium

Copper is a co-factor of many enzymes and plays an important role in energy metabolism and the formation of erythrocytes and connective tissue. There is no established RDA for copper but its estimated safe and adequate daily dietary intake (ESADDI) is 1.5–3.0 mg. The main dietary sources of copper are shown in Table 7.2. Intake of up to 10 mg/day is known to be safe and toxicity from dietary copper ingestion is extremely rare, but athletes who take zinc supplements may compromise the gastrointestinal absorption of copper due to the similar physicochemical properties of these two minerals. Athletes should be aware that large doses of Vitamin C can also limit copper absorption.[34]

The effects of copper deficiency on immune function include impaired antibody formation, inflammatory response, phagocytic killing power, NKCA, and lymphocyte stimulation responses.[2, 8, 10] The results of changes in copper status due to exercise and training are controversial, and perhaps reflect the inadequacy of techniques used to measure copper status, or a redistribution of copper between body compartments, although athletes have been reported to lose copper in sweat collected after exercise.[72] Compared with sedentary controls, several groups of athletes have been found to have similar or higher resting blood levels of copper.[73–75] Thus, the copper status of athletes seems to be normal. Following an acute bout of prolonged exercise, the plasma copper concentration may rise[76, 77] or remain unchanged.[13] Dressendorfer et al. [48] reported a substantial increase in plasma copper concentration during the first 8 days of a 20-day road race and this elevation persisted for the remainder of the race. This was attributed to an increase in the production of ceruloplasmin by the liver[48] as part of the acute-phase response. Ceruloplasmin is a glycoprotein that binds copper and is thought to exert a protective effect against cellular damage caused by free radicals.

The RDA for selenium is 70 μg for males and 55 μg for females (Table 7.2). Selenium deficiency can affect all components of the immune system.[2] Selenium functions as an antioxidant and is also a co-factor of glutathione peroxidase/reductase and thus influences the quenching of ROS. Selenium plays a synergistic role with vitamin E to protect cell membranes from free-radical damage. Because exercise increases free-radical production and lipid peroxidation, it is possible that the requirement of selenium is increased in those individuals involved in a regular intensive training program. Increased degranulation of blood neutrophils occurs during exercise and the elevated activity of the granular enzymes such as myeloperoxidase in the circulation may be one of the causes of increased free-radical damage.[78] However, any selenium supplement should be taken with caution; supplements of amounts up to the RDA appear nontoxic, yet the safety of larger doses has not been confirmed and intakes of 25 mg (approximately 40 x RDA) have been associated with vomiting, abdominal pain, hair loss, and fatigue.[34]

At present, there is no information on the dietary intake of selenium in athletes. Although further research is required, it is likely that both copper and selenium requirements are increased during heavy training. However, given that the diet of the general population in the Western world is adequate in selenium and excessive intake of selenium can be harmful, there is no scientific justification for recommending selenium supplements.

7.4.3 Manganese, Cobalt, and Fluorine

Manganese is a co-factor of the enzyme superoxide dismutase, which aids in protection against free radicals.[79] The RDA for manganese is 2.0–5.0 mg/day. Sources are whole grain products, dried peas and beans, leafy vegetables and bananas. The effects of exercise on manganese status are presently unknown, but training is associated with an increase in levels of antioxidant enzymes, suggesting there may be an increased requirement for manganese during periods of increased training. As with other trace elements it is also likely that losses of manganese in urine and sweat will be higher in athletes than nonathletes.

Cobalt, as a component of Vitamin B12, promotes the development of red and white blood cells in the bone marrow.[80] Deficiencies are associated with pernicious anemia, reduced blood leukocyte count, impaired lymphocyte proliferation and impaired bactericidal capacity of neutrophils.[81, 82] Major food sources of cobalt are meat, liver, and milk. Hence, athletes who avoid animal foods are at risk of developing cobalt/B12 deficiency.

Although not directly required for normal immune function, fluorine is needed for the normal formation of healthy bones and teeth and protects against dental caries (tooth decay by oral bacteria).[83, 84] Given the relatively high intake of sugary foods and sports drinks by athletes,[14,54] good oral hygiene is important to maintain healthy teeth. Frequent intakes of carbohydrates–particularly sugars–will repeatedly depress the Stephan curve below the critical pH with a resultant net demineralization of the teeth. 85 It is therefore essential that all sports people maintain good plaque control. The RDA for fluorine is 1.5–4.0 mg/day, and this trace element is found in milk, egg yolk, seafood and drinking water. Several toothpastes and mouthrinses contain fluorine (as sodium fluoride) and in some countries fluoride is added to drinking water. Excess intake of fluoride is poisonous due to its inhibitory effects on a number of enzymes, including some of the enzymes of glycolysis.

Table 7.4 Sports at Risk for Marginal Mineral Nutrition

Diet or condition	Sports at risk
Low body weight–chronically low energy intakes to achieve low body weight	Gymnastics, jockeying, ballet, ice dancing, dancing
Making competition weight–drastic weight loss regimen to achieve desired weight category	Weight class sports (rowing, wrestling, boxing, judo)
Low fat–drastic weight loss to achieve low body fat	Body building
Vegetarian diets	Endurance athletes
Training in hot humid climate	Endurance athletes

7.5 CONCLUSIONS

There are several minerals that exert a modulatory role on immune function; likewise, there are several minerals deemed important for optimal exercise performance. Zinc and iron, and to a certain extent, magnesium, selenium, and copper, fall into both categories. Deficiencies in these minerals are generally detrimental to immune function, although a mild deficiency in iron may exert a protective mechanism against bacterial infection by withholding iron from invading micro-organisms, thus limiting their proliferation. In most athletes, the dietary intake of these nutrients is at least as much as (and usually more than) that of the general population, although the athlete's mineral requirement may be increased by a heavy training schedule, particularly in hot weather. Deficiencies can be exacerbated by unbalanced diets, e.g., diets rich in fiber and refined carbohydrates (limited zinc absorption), vegetarian diets (likely to be low in heme-iron, zinc, and cobalt content) or restricted-energy diets when athletes are trying to lose body weight (Table 7.4 highlights those sports in which athletes are at risk of inadequate mineral nutrition). Supplements must be taken with caution, however, as in all cases, ingesting excessive amounts of iron, copper, selenium, or zinc can be at least as harmful as ingesting too little.

Both heavy exercise and nutrition exert separate influences on immune function; these influences appear to be greater when exercise stress and poor nutrition act synergistically. Exercise training increases the body's requirement for most nutrients, including trace elements and, in many cases, these increased needs are countered by increased food consumption. However, some athletes adopt an unbalanced dietary regimen in the mistaken belief that it will confer a performance advantage and many surveys show that few athletes follow the best dietary pattern for optimal sport nutrition. Many athletes routinely take nutrient supplements that, if not needed, may do more harm than good. In view of this, athletes are advised to consult a qualified sports nutritionist to assess their nutritional status and needs before taking large amounts of (probably) unnecessary supplements.

7.6 SUMMARY

Some minerals have an essential role in the functioning of immune cells. Minerals are classified as macrominerals or microminerals (trace elements), based on the extent of their occurrence in the body. Of particular importance here are the trace elements that each compose less than 0.001% of total body mass, of which 14 have been identified as essential for maintenance of health. Several minerals are known to exert modulatory effects on immune function, including iron, zinc, copper, selenium, and magnesium, and deficiencies of one or more of these minerals are associated with immune dysfunction and increased incidence of infection. Regular exercise, particularly in a hot environment, incurs increased losses of these minerals in sweat and urine, which means that the daily requirement is increased in athletes engaged in heavy training. However, provided the athlete is consuming a well-balanced diet that meets the daily energy requirement, the intake of minerals will be more than adequate to offset the increased requirements. Supplements are not usually needed and should be discouraged, since excess intakes of most trace elements can interfere with the absorption of other trace elements, have toxic effects, or inhibit the immune system.

With the exception of iron and zinc, isolated deficiencies of trace elements are rare. Supplements are generally not needed unless fresh meat, fruit, and vegetables are not readily available; the athlete is a vegetarian; or is restricting energy intake in order to lose body weight or maintain a low body weight. The presence of diarrhea, use of diuretics, excessive alcohol intake and eating disorders may also contribute to the development of a deficiency state that could be remedied by appropriate mineral supplements—i.e., not more than the daily recommended dietary allowance.

REFERENCES

1. Chandra, R.K., Nutrition and the immune system: An introduction, *Am. J. Clin. Nutr.,* 66, 460S, 1997.
2. Scrimshaw, N.S., and SanGiovanni, J.P., Synergism of nutrition, infection and immunity: an overview, *Am. J. Clin. Nutr.,* 66, 464S, 1997.
3. Scrimshaw, N.S., and Young, V.R., The requirements of human nutrition, *Sci. Am.,* 235(3), 50, 1976.
4. Dreisen, S., Nutrition and the immune response–a review, *Int. J. Vitamin Nutr. Res.,* 49, 220, 1978.
5. Chandra, R.K., Nutrition and immunity: lessons from the past and new insights into the future, *Am. J. Clin. Nutr.,* 53, 1087, 1991.
6. O'Leary, M.J., and Coakley, J.H., Nutrition and immunonutrition, *Br. J. Anaesth,* 77(1), 118, 1996.
7. Mertz, W., The essential trace elements, *Science,* 213, 1332, 1981.
8. Sherman, A.R., Zinc, copper and iron nutriture and immunity, *J. Nutr.,* 122, 604, 1992.
9. Dallman, P.R., Iron deficiency and the immune response, *Am. J. Clin. Nutr.,* 46, 329, 1987.
10. Lukasewycz, O.A., and Prohaska, J.R., The immune response in copper deficiency, *Ann. NY Acad. Sci.,* 587, 147, 1990.

11. Haymes, F.M. and Lamanca, J.J., Iron loss in runners during exercise: implications and recommendations, *Sports Med.,* 7, 277, 1989.

12. Clarkson, P.M., Minerals: exercise performance and supplementation in athletes, in *Foods, Nutrition and Sports Performance,* Williams, C., Devlin, J., Eds., E. & F.N. Spon, London, 1992, 113.

13. Anderson, R.A., Polansky, M.M., and Bryden, N.A., Strenuous running: Acute effects on chromium, copper, zinc and selected clinical variables in urine and serum of male runners, *Biol. Trace Elem. Res.,* 6, 327, 1984.

14. Brouns, F., *Nutritional Needs of Athletes.* Wiley, Chichester, 1993.

15. Gleeson, M., Fluid and micronutrient intake: needs for physical activity, *Brit. J. Therap. Rehab.,* 4, 252, 1997.

16. Puschmann, M. and Ganzoni, A.M., Increased resistance of iron-deficient mice to salmonella infection, *Infect. Immun,* 17, 663, 1997.

17. Dufaux, B., Hoederath, A., Streitberger, I., Hollmann, W., and Assman, G., Serum ferritin, transferrin, haptoglobin, and iron in middle- and long-distance runners, elite rowers, and professional racing cyclists, *Int. J. Sports Med.,* 2, 43, 1981.

18. Eichner, E.R., Sports anemia, iron supplements and blood doping, *Med. Sci. Sports Exerc.,* 24, S315, 1992.

19. Deakin, V., Iron deficiency in athletes: identification, prevention and dietary treatment, in. *Clinical Sports Nutrition,* Burke, L. and Deakin, V., Eds., McGraw-Hill, Sydney, 1994, 175.

20. Blum, S.M., Sherman, A.R., and Boileau, R.A., The effects of fitness-type exercise on iron status in adult women, *Am. J. Clin. Nutr.,* 43, 456, 1986.

21. Magazanik, A., Weinstein, Y., Dlin, R.A., Derin, M., Schwartzman, S., and Allalouf, D., Iron deficiency caused by 7 weeks of intensive physical exercise, *Eur. J. Appl. Physiol.,* 57, l98, 1998.

22. Pattini, A., Schena, F., and Guidi, G.C., Serum ferritin and serum iron changes after cross-country and roller ski endurance races, *Eur J. Appl. Physiol.,* 61, 55, 1990.

23. Goldblum, S.E., Cohen, D.A., Jay, M., and McClain, C.J., Interleukin 1-induced depression of iron and zinc: role of granulocytes and lactoferrin, *Am. J. Physiol.,* 252, E27, 1987.

24. Ullum, H., Haahr, P.M., Diamant, M., Palmo, J., Halkjaer-Kristensen, J., and Pedersen, B.K., Bicycle exercise enhances plasma 1L-6 but does not change IL-Iα, IL-1β, IL-6, or TNFα pre-mRNA in BMNC, *J. Appl. Physiol.,* 77, 93, 1994.

25. Bruunsgaard, H., Galbo, H., Halkjaer-Kristensen, J., Johansen, T.L., MacLean, D.A., and Pedersen, B.K., Exercise-induced increase in serum interleukin-6 in humans is related to muscle damage, *J. Physiol.,* 499(3), 833, 1997.

26. Galan, P., Thibault, H., Preziosi, P., and Herchberg, S., Interleukin-2 production in iron-deficient children, *Biol. Trace Elem. Res.,* 32, 421, 1992.

27. Ascherio, A., Willett, W.C., Rimm, E.B., Giovannucci, E.L., and Stampfer, M.J., Dietary iron intake and risk of coronary disease among men, *Circulation,* 89, 969, 1994.

28. Konig, D., Weinstock, C., Keul, J., Northoff, H., and Berg, A., Zinc, iron and magnesium status in athletes–influence on the regulation of exercise-induced stress and immune function, *Exerc. Immun. Rev.,* Human Kinetics, Champaign IL, USA, 1998, 4, 2.

29. Cardier, J.E., Romano, E., and Soyano, A., T-lymphocytes subsets in experimental iron overload, *Immunopharm. Immunotoxicol.,* 19, 75, 1997.

30. Cunningham-Rundles, S., Effects of nutritional status on immunological function, *Am. J. Clin. Nutr.,* 35, 1202, 1982.

31. Helyar, L., and Sherman, A.R., Iron deficiency and interleukin-1 production by rat leukocytes, *Am. J. Clin. Nutr.,*46, 343, 1987.
32. Shephard, R.J., and Shek, P.N., Heavy exercise, nutrition and immune function: is there a connection? *Int. J. Sports Med.,* 16(8), 491, 1995.
33. van Asbeck, S., Marx, J.J.M., Struvenberg, A., van Kats, J.H., and Verhoet, J., Effect of iron (III) in the presence of various ligands on the phagocytic and metabolic activity of human polymorphonuclear leukocytes, *J. Immunol.,* 132, 851, 1994.
34. Williams, M.H., *Nutrition for Fitness and Sport*, 4th edition, McGraw-Hill, New York, 1995.
35. Deuster, P.A., Day, B.A., Singh, A., Douglass, L., and Moser-Veillon, P.B., Zinc status of highly trained women runners and untrained women, *Am. J. Clin. Nutr.,* 49, 1295, 1989.
36. Ricci, G., Masotti, M., De Paoli Vitali, E., Vedovato, M., and Zanotti, G., Effects of exercise on haematological parameters, serum iron, serum ferritin, red cell 2,3-diphosphoglycerate and creatine contents, and serum erythropoietin in long-distance runners during basal training, *Acta. Haematol.,* 80, 95, 1988.
37. Erp-Baart, A.M.J. van, Saris, W.H.M., Binkhorst, R.A., and Elvers, J.W.H., Nation-wide survey on nutritional habits in elite athletes, part II. Mineral and vitamin intake, *Int. J. Sports Med.,*10, S11, 1989.
38. Fogelholm, M., Vitamins, minerals and supplementation in soccer, *J. Sports Sci.,*12, S23, 1994.
39. Emery, T., *Iron and Your Health,* CRC, Boca Raton, 1991.
40. Fairbanks, V., Iron in medicine and nutrition, in *Modern Nutrition in Health and Disease*, Shils, M., Ed., Lea and Febiger, Philadelphia, 1994.
41. Singh, A., Failla, M.L., and Deuster, P.A., Exercise-induced changes in immune function: effects of zinc supplementation, *J. Appl. Physiol.,* 76, 2298, 1994.
42. Cunningham, B.C., Bass, S., Fuh, G., and Wells, J.A., Zinc mediation of the binding of human growth hormone to the human prolactin receptor, *Science,* 250, 1709, 1990.
43. Prasad, A.S., Zinc: An overview, *Nutr,*11, 93, 1995.
44. Bettger, W.J., and O'Dell, B.L., A critical physiological role of zinc in the structure and function of biomembranes, *Life Sci.,* 28, 1425, 1991.
45. Chvapil, M., Stankova, L., Zukoski, C. IV., and Zukoski, C. III., Inhibition of some functions of polymorphonuclear leukocytes by *in vitro* zinc, *J. Lab Clin Med,* 89(1), 135, 1977.
46. Ogino, K., Izumi, Y., Segawa, H., Takeyama, Y., Ishiyama, H., Houbara, T., Uda, T., and Yamashita, S., Zinc hydroxide induced respiratory burst in rat neutrophils, *Eur J. Pharmacol,* 270, 73, 1994.
47. Prasad, A.S., Marginal deficiency of zinc and immunological effects, *Prog. Clin. Biol. Res,* 380, 1, 1993.
48. Dressendorfer, R.H., Wade, C.E., Keen, C.L., and Scaff, J.H., Plasma mineral levels in marathon runners during a 20-day road race, *Physician Sportsmed,* 10, 113, 1982.
49. Ohno, H., Yamashita, K., and Doi, R., Exercise-induced changes in blood zinc and related proteins in humans, *J. Appl Physiol,* 58(5), 1453, 1985.

50. Lukaski, H.C., Bolonchuk, W.W., Klevay, L.M., Milne, D.B., and Sandstead, H.H., Changes in plasma zinc content after exercise in men fed a low-zinc diet, *Am. J. Physiol.*, 247, E88, 1984.

51. Ruz, M., Cavan, K.R., Bettger, W.J., and Gibson, R.S., Erythrocytes, erythrocyte membranes, neutrophils and platelets as biopsy materials for the assessment of zinc status in humans, *Br. J. Nutr.*, 68, 515, 1992.

52. Robson, P.J., Blannin, A.K., Gleeson, M., Walsh, N.P., and Clark, A.M., The effects of intermittent high intensity exercise on blood zinc status and urinary zinc excretion, *J. Sports Sci.*, 16, 59, 1998.

53. Dressendorfer, R.H., and Sockolov, R., Hypozincemia in runners, *Physician Sportsmed.*, 8, 97, 1980.

54. Hawley, J.A., Dennis, S.C., Lindsey, F.H., and Noakes, T.D., Nutritional practices of athletes: are they sub-optimal? *J. Sports Sci.* 13, S75, 1995.

55. Haralambic, G., Serum zinc in athletes in training, *Int. J. Sports Med.*, 2, 135, 1981.

56. Solomons, N.W., On the assessment of zinc and copper nutriture in man, *Am. J. Clin. Nutr.*, 32, 856, 1979.

57. Pilch, S.M., and Senti, F.R., Analysis of zinc data from the second national health and nutrition examination survey (NHANES II), *J. Nutr.*, 115, 1393, 1985.

58. Black, R.E., Therapeutic and preventative effects of zinc on serious childhood infectious diseases in developing countries, *Am. J. Clin. Nutr.*, 68(2 Suppl), 476S, 1998.

59. Chandra, R.K., Excessive intake of zinc impairs immune responses, *JAMA*, 252, 1443, 1984.

60. Sunzel, B., Holm, S., Reuterving, C.-O., Soderberg, T., Hallmans, G., and Hanstrom, L., The effect of zinc on bacterial phagocytosis, killing and cytoprotection in human polymorphonuclear leukocytes, *APMIS*, 103(9), 635, 1995.

61. Spencer, H., and Osis, D., Studies on magnesium metabolism in men: Original data and review, *Magnesium*, 7, 271, 1988.

62. Wacker, W.E.C., and Parisi, A.F., Magnesium metabolism, *New Eng. J. Med.*, 278, 658, 1968.

63. Bilbey, D.L., and Prabhakaran, V.M., Muscle cramps and magnesium deficiency: Case reports, *Can. Fam. Physician*, 42, 1348, 1996.

64. Casoni, I., Guglielmini, C., Graziano, L., Reali, M.G., Mazzotta, D., and Abbasciano, V., Changes of magnesium concentrations in endurance athletes, *Int. J. Sports Med.*, 11, 234, 1990.

65. Cordova, A., and Alvarez-Mon, M., Behavior of zinc in physical exercise: A special reference to immunity and fatigue, *Neurosci. Biobehav. Res.*, 19, 439, 1995.

66. Deuster, P.A., Dolev, E., Kyle, S.B., Anderson, R.A., and Schoomaker, E.B., Magnesium homeostasis during high-intensity anaerobic exercise in men, *J. Appl. Physiol.*, 62, 545, 1987.

67. Kelepouris, E., Kasama, R., and Agus, Z.S., Effects of intracellular magnesium on calcium, potassium and chloride channels, *Mineral Electrolyte Metab.*, 19, 277, 1993.

68. Rock, E., Astier, C., Lab, C., Vignon, X., Gueux, E., Motta, C., and Rayssiguier, Y., Dietary magnesium deficiency in rats enhances free radical production in skeletal muscle, *J. Nutr.*, 125, 1205, 1995.

69. Zhu, Z., Kimura, M., and Itokawa, Y., Selenium concentration and glutathione per-
    oxidase activity in selenium and magnesium deficient rats, *Biol. Trace Elem. Res.,*
    37, 209, 1993.
70. Kurantsin-Mills, J., Cassidy, M.M., Stafford, R.E., and Weglicki, W.B., Marked alter-
    ations in circulating inflammatory cells during cardiomyopathy development in a
    magnesium-deficient rat model, *Br. J. Nutr.,* 78, 845, 1997.
71. Weglicki, W.B., Dickens, B.F., Wagner, T.L., Chmielinska, J.J., and Phillips, T.M.,
    Immunoregulation by neuropeptides in magnesium deficiency: Ex vivo effect of
    enhanced substance-P production on circulating T-lymphocytes from magnesium-
    deficient mice, *Magnes. Res.,* 9, 3, 1996.
72. Gutteridge, J.M.C., Rowley, D.A., and Halliwell, B., Copper and iron complexes
    catalytic for oxygen radical reactions in sweat from human athletes, *Clin. Chim. Acta.,*
    145, 167, 1995.
73. Lukaski, H.C., Bolonchuk, W.W., Klevay, L.M., Milne, D.B., and Sandstead, H.H.,
    Maximum oxygen consumption as related to magnesium, copper and zinc nutriture,
    Am. J. Clin. Nutr., 37, 407, 1983.
74. Lukaski, H.C., Effects of exercise training on human copper and zinc nutrition, *Adv.
    Exp. Med. Biol.,* 258, 163, 1989.
75. Weight, L.M., Noakes, T.D., Labadarios, D., Graves, J., Jacobs, P., and Berman, P.A.,
    Vitamin and mineral status of trained athletes including the effects of supplementation,
    Am. J. Clin. Nutr., 47, 186, 1988.
76. Ohno H., Yahata, T., Hirata, F., Yamamura, K., Doi, R., Harada, M., and Taniguchi,
    N., Changes in dopamine-Beta-hydroxylase, and copper, and catecholamine concen-
    trations in human plasma with physical exercise, *J. Sports Med.,* 24, 315, 1984.
77. Olha, A.E., Klissouras, V., Sullivan, J.D., and Skoryna, S.C., Effect of exercise on
    concentration of elements in the serum, *J. Sports Med.,* 22, 414, 1982.
78. Gleeson, M., and Bishop, N.C., Immunology, in *Basic and Applied Sciences for Sports
    Medicine,* Maughan, R.J., Ed., Butterworth Heinemann, Oxford, 199, 1999.
79. Christianson, D.W., Structural chemistry and biology of manganese metalloenzymes.
    Prog. Biophys. Molec. Biol., 67(2–3), 217, 1997.
80. Solomon, E.P., Schmidt, R.R., and Adragna, P.J., *Human Anatomy and Physiology,*
    Second edition, Saunders, Philadelphia, 651, 1991.
81. Nauss, K.M., and Newberne, P.M., Effects of dietary folate, vitamin B12 and methion-
    ine/choline deficiency on immune function, *Adv. Exp. Med. Biol.,* 135, 63, 1981.
82. Beisel, W.R., Edelman, R., Nauss, K., and Suskind, R.M., Single nutrient effects on
    immunologic functions, *JAMA,* 245, 53, 1981.
83. Position of the American Dietetic Association: the impact of fluoride on dental health,
    J. Am. Dietetic Assoc., 94(12), 1428, 1994.
84. Bowen, W.H., The role of fluoride toothpastes in the prevention of dental caries, *J.
    Royal Soc. Med.,* 88(9), 505, 1995.
85. Milosevic, A., Dental health and the serious athlete, *Good Dietary Practice News,* 9,
    6, 1992.

CHAPTER 8

Cancer, Nutrition, and Exercise Immunology

Jeffrey A. Woods

CONTENTS

8.1 INTRODUCTION

In the United States, about 560,000 people are expected to die of cancer this year. Although cancer is the second leading cause of death behind heart disease, death rates from heart disease are in dramatic decline, whereas those of some specific cancers are rising.[1] In 1972, President Nixon declared "war on cancer," and while no global cure has been found, much progress has been made in detecting and treating cancer. This has led to longer survival times in those afflicted with the disease. Its financial costs remain great both to the individual and to society.

It has been suggested that cancer is a largely preventable disease. Although genetics (particularly mutations in the p53 tumor suppressor gene) are a factor in the development of cancer, contraction of the disease cannot be explained entirely by heredity. Behaviors such as tobacco and alcohol use, improper diet, and lack of physical activity have a profound impact on the risk of developing cancer. Indeed, it has been suggested that approximately 30% to 60% of all cancers could be prevented if people adopted a healthier lifestyle including proper diet and physical activity.[2] This chapter will discuss human epidemiological and animal experimental data regarding the role of exercise/physical activity and diet in reducing cancer incidence and progression. Where possible, it will focus on the potential role of selected dietary factors and exercise in modulating anti-tumor immune defense mechanisms.

8.2 IMMUNE MECHANISMS RESPONSIBLE FOR CANCER DEFENSE

Many lines of evidence are consistent with the idea that cancer is not a single disease, nor are its causes one dimensional. Substantial evidence indicates that human cancers are the result of multiple sequential mutations that ultimately lead to uncontrolled cell growth. Perhaps the most devastating aspect of cancer is that it can spread or metastasize to sites external to the original site of growth. The immune system is one of the body's major defense mechanisms against the outbreak and control of malignant cells. Immune surveillance of neoplastic cells is effective against the development of several virally induced cancers but does not seem to play a role in preventing the development of most forms induced by physical or chemical carcinogens.[3] However, this lack of surveillance against spontaneous or carcinogenic tumors does not mean that these types of tumors are not sensitive to immunological defenses once established. Indeed, many altered cancer cells express antigens that can be recognized as foreign by the host immune system.[4] Successful tumors (i.e. those that spread) typically arise spontaneously and tend to be less immunogenic than those that are induced by viral or carcinogenic insult.[5] Given that the immune system is important in the control of cancer outbreak and spread, the following section will briefly describe several immune-effector mechanisms involved in cancer defense. One theme that is apparent is that, due to the diversity of different types of cancer, different immune-effector mechanisms play different roles in the destruction of cancers cells in different experimental tumor models. In other words, there is no one single important immune defense mechanism capable of fighting the myriad forms of cancer.

8.2.1   Lymphocytes and Antibodies

B lymphocytes are cells derived from the bone marrow that ultimately produce soluble protein antibodies that have exquisite specificity for certain protein antigens, like those that can be differentially expressed on tumor cells. Theoretically, antibodies can specifically bind to tumor cells and promote their destruction through the activation of complement and antibody-dependent cellular cytotoxicity (ADCC) performed by macrophages (Mϕs), natural killer (NK) cells, or neutrophils. Mϕs can also phagocytose and destroy antibody-coated tumor cells.[6]

Unfortunately, while there are occasional successes in the treatment of various cancers with specific antibodies,[7] in most instances a strong antibody response to tumor antigens does not seem to correlate with improved resistance of the host to tumors.[8, 9] The reasons for this are unclear but are likely related to tumor escape mechanisms including antigenic modulation, lack of immunogenicity, or antigen shedding.[6] Despite the murky role of the *in vivo* antibody response in cancer protection, many novel approaches to anti-tumor therapy have adopted specific anti-tumor antibodies.[10]

8.2.2   Natural and Lymphokine-Activated Killer Cells

Natural killer (NK) cells consist of a sub-population of lymphocytes that can kill certain tumor cells without prior sensitization and without the requirement for major histocompatability complex (MHC) restriction. In initial studies, NK cells were found to lack most of the markers and properties of T and B cells.[11] Over time, NK cells were found to represent a third and distinct population of lymphocytes (about 10%–15% in human peripheral blood) in addition to T and B lymphocytes, expressing a characteristic set of markers (CD3-, CD2+, CD16+, and CD56+).[12] Lymphokine-activated killer (LAK) cells are generated when NK cells are exposed to cytokines such as IL-2, IL-12, or interferon. LAK cells can kill a wider variety of tumor cells than NK cells and do so more efficiently.

Observations that are consistent with (but do not necessarily prove) an *in vivo* role for NK cells in anti-tumor defense include the finding of increased spontaneous tumors in animals at an age when endogenous NK cell activity falls, the ability of T cell-deficient nude mice to reject some tumors, a reduction in NK cell activity in certain cancer patients, and increased tumor metastasis in mice experimentally depleted of NK cells using anti-NK cell antibodies.[6]

8.2.3   T Lymphocytes

T cells, derived from the thymus gland, are theoretically important in cell-mediated immunity against tumors by recognition of tumor-specific antigens. It is well known that T cells are of critical importance for the rejection of virally and chemically induced tumors that express high levels of non-self antigens,[6] however, spontaneously arising tumors are low in immunogenicity. There has been limited success in the treatment of some forms of cancer using adoptive transfer of tumor-specific T cells activated and expanded with IL-2.[13]

8.2.4   Macrophages

Mφs are potent, non-specific immune cells that, when activated by specific signals (i.e., interferon-γ, lipopolysaccharide), can readily lyse various tumor cells. The cytolytic or cytostatic effects of Mφs on tumor cells involves cell–cell contact and/or the secretion of a number of distinct toxic molecules (i.e., tumor necrosis factor, nitric oxide), but phagocytosis and subsequent killing of ingested tumor cells is also of importance. Mφs can also act in concert with antibodies in performing ADCC. Because of the rather selective killing of tumor- and not normal host cells by Mφs, the role of this cell in immunosurveillance and immunotherapy has been examined. At present, there is no irrefutable evidence to establish the notion that Mφs destroy tumor cells in early stages of cancer.[14] However, there is evidence that suggests that activation of Mφs *in vivo* with biological response modifiers (i.e., BCG, *P. acnes*) and adoptive transfer of Mφs activated *in vitro* can eliminate or reduce cancer and metastasis in some models.[15]

8.3 EPIDEMIOLOGICAL STUDIES ON EXERCISE AND SELECTED DIETARY FACTORS IN THE PREVENTION OF CANCER

This section will briefly review the literature regarding the epidemiological evidence linking exercise and selected dietary factors to all-cause cancer mortality and site-specific cancer incidence rates. A more detailed analysis and discussion can be found in several excellent reviews.[16–24]

8.3.1   Exercise/Physical Activity

There has been a recent explosion in the number of epidemiological studies examining the association between physical activity and cancer incidence and mortality. Most studies have shown that physical activity as assessed directly by subjective recall, job classification, former athletic status, or indirectly by physical fitness, is inversely related to the incidence of and mortality from cancer. The strengths of the associations vary, depending on the site of the cancer, with several studies documenting no association.

The most consistent and strongest relationship between physical activity and cancer incidence/mortality has been shown for cancer of the colon. Despite a few exceptions,[25–27] the overwhelming majority of studies support the hypothesis that greater occupational activity[28–34] or participation in exercise[35–37] are protective against the development of colon cancer. This effect is substantial, leading to a 50%–100% greater risk in inactive than in physically active groups. The amount of physical activity needed to ensure protection is unclear. However, several studies have evidence for a clear dose–response relationship.[28, 30, 36, 34]

At least 13 studies have examined the association between physical activity and breast cancer incidence. The study designs, subjects, and findings vary, but, despite these differences, 10 of the 13 studies have demonstrated a decreased risk of breast cancer for women who had higher daily energy expenditures or physically demanding jobs, or who engaged in athletics while in college.[19] The magnitude of the effect, while not as strong as that for physical activity and colon cancer, is still significant; inactive women are 10%–60% more likely to develop breast cancer than active women.[17] What is controversial is the amount and timing of the physical activity/exercise needed to protect against breast cancer.[38, 39] Unfortunately, an underlying problem is that most studies have failed to quantify the amount and timing of physical activity accurately in relation to the measurement period.

Cancers at others sites are also inversely related to level of physical activity. However, the consistency and strengths of the associations tend to be lower than those for colon and breast cancer. Women with occupations demanding a low level of physical activity had an increased risk of cancer of the corpus uteri and ovary than those with jobs demanding a high level of physical activity.[40] In another study, physically active women had a 50% lower risk for the development of endometrial cancer, but with no evidence of a dose–response relationship.[41] The association between physical activity and prostate cancer has been examined and in 9 of 17 studies an inverse relationship has been observed.[20] For example, physically active Harvard alumni who expended (>16.8MJ/wk^{-1}) accurately when assessed both in the 1960's and in 1977 had a greatly reduced relative risk (i.e., RR = 0.12) when compared with inactive counterparts (<4.2MJ/wk^{-1}).[42] However, in 3 of the 17 studies, physical activity was associated with an increased risk of prostate cancer.[20] In the few available studies regarding lung cancer, inactive people have been found to be between 20%–50% more likely to develop lung cancer after adjustment for smoking and several other confounders. With the exception of one study,[43] the risks of cancer at other sites, including bladder, stomach, and pancreas have revealed no significant associations with physical activity.[26, 44, 45] Unfortunately, because of the limited number of studies and the weak associations, it is hard to make conclusive statements regarding the interaction between physical activity and these site-specific cancers. The inconsistencies in some studies and the lack of dose-dependent relationships in most studies are likely related to the imprecise measurement of physical activity.

8.3.2 Diet

Many human epidemiological studies suggest that most cancer deaths are attributable to lifestyle, including nutritional factors, tobacco use, and alcohol consumption. Nutrients and non-nutrient dietary components probably account for a large percentage of colon, breast, and prostate cancers.[16]

Diets with especially high-fat and low-fiber content are generally associated with increased risk for developing colon cancer.[46] The type of fat is also an important factor. Relative to saturated fats from red meats, mortality from colon cancer is lower in areas where poly- or monounsaturated olive oil and fish oils are consumed.[47] Because diets high in fat are also high in calories, and because total caloric intake is also related to cancer incidence, it is hard to separate whether the effects of these diets are due to changes in specific types of fats in the diet or to an increased total number of calories. Experimental animal studies should help clear up this dilemma. A recent examination provided substantive evidence that the intake of fiber-rich foods is inversely related to colon cancer risk.[48] These data implied that the risk of colon cancer could be reduced by 31% if fiber intake could be increased to 25 g/day.

The role of dietary factors in breast cancer development is a bit more confused. Experimental animal studies and international correlations with breast cancer mortality and fat intake by humans provide evidence for a tumor-promoting effect.[49] In contrast, several cohort studies have failed to demonstrate lower breast cancer risk in women who consume low-fat diets.[50] As was the case with colon cancer, the type of fat may also play a role with intake of long chain n-3 polyunsaturated, monounsaturated, and short- and medium-chain saturated fats associated with lower breast cancer mortality relative to high intakes of n-6 essential fatty acids.[51] However, one difficulty in interpreting the findings of most epidemiological studies is that most do not accurately assess or take into account the relative levels of different fatty acids compared with the total amount of fat consumed.

International comparisons show the same positive correlation between prostate cancer mortality rates and fat intake that exist for breast cancer. Indeed, the case-control studies support the association and some have even demonstrated dose–response effects.[21] Unfortunately, the contribution of individual fatty acids to prostate cancer protection or promotion is unclear.

Vitamins have long been of interest to cancer researchers because of their roles in growth, development, carcinogen metabolism, and as antioxidants. High dietary intakes of vitamins A, C, and E have been most associated with low incidence rates for cancer.[52] However, it has been hard to delineate whether the actual intake of these vitamins is important or if the intake of other nutrients in foods that typically contain these vitamins (i.e., vegetables and fruits) is responsible for the protective effect against cancer. There is little evidence that consuming vitamin supplements above and beyond that obtained through a proper diet prevents cancer. Indeed, the recommendation has been that consumption of foods rich in vitamins and not the use of supplements be the goal of a proper diet.

With numerous reports having found inverse relationships between vegetable consumption and gastrointestinal tract cancer,[54] and some having found inverse relationships to lung, breast, and prostate cancers,[53] epidemiological evidence has provided circumstantial evidence for cancer prevention by dietary vegetables and fruits.[53] Studies such as these have led to an explosion in research aimed at defining the non-nutrient chemical constituents in the foods that are responsible. Among some that have shown the most promise as inhibitors of cancer include indoles, isothiocyanates, flavonoids, lycopene and carotenoids.[53] It is still too early to tell, however, whether these factors are important in reducing incidence rates of various forms of cancer.

8.4   EXPERIMENTAL STUDIES ON THE INFLUENCE OF EXERCISE AND SELECTED DIETARY FACTORS ON CANCER INCIDENCE AND PROGRESSION AND ANTI-TUMOR IMMUNE DEFENSES

Although many potential mechanisms can be attributed to link dietary factors and exercise with cancer incidence and progression, one link may involve the modulation of various components of anti-tumor immune defense by diet and exercise. The section below includes a brief overview of experimental studies examining the influence of selected dietary factors and exercise on cancer incidence and progression and anti-tumor immune defenses.

8.4.1   Animal Studies Regarding Exercise and Cancer Incidence and Progression

Another approach to the study of exercise and cancer has been the utilization of experimental animal models. Studies of this nature clearly have merits, in that the influence of genetics, diet, dose of carcinogen or tumor load, and other confounding factors can be controlled. Furthermore, important questions about physiological significance and biological mechanism(s) can be addressed. However, there are obvious difficulties in attempting to extrapolate findings to spontaneous human tumors. Typically these studies have examined the relationship between forced or voluntary exercise and the growth of transplantable, chemically induced, and/or spontaneous tumors in rodents. Many of these studies have reported some beneficial effect of exercise on tumor incidence or progression. However, in general, the studies have been descriptive in nature and have failed to offer plausible biological mechanisms as to how exercise might influence neoplasia.

Almost without exception, early animal studies reported that exercise inhibited tumor growth in transplantable tumor systems[55, 56] or tumor occurrence in chemically induced or spontaneous tumor models.[57–59] Unfortunately, interpretation of these early studies is confounded by the fact that the animals were subjected to large amounts of forced exercise. For example, Rusch and Kline (1944) subjected their mice to 18 h of daily exercise in rotating drums and documented a reduction in tumor growth vs. control animals. A primary concern in the interpretation of these early data has been whether exercise exerted an effect independent of its effect on normal maturation, energy intake, and body composition, the last two variables being strongly linked to tumorigenesis.[60] In these early studies, two theories were advanced to account for the tumor-inhibiting effect of exercise. One was that tumor cells were less likely to develop or continue to grow if there was little or no excess food energy available.[56] Indeed, this contention is supported by studies in which dietary restriction decreased tumor incidence and progression.[61] However, restriction of energy intake also improves anti-tumor immune defenses.[62] The other theory was that fatigued muscles produced a factor that inhibited tumor growth.[55] Although an intriguing concept, there has never been any documentation regarding this latter hypothesis.

In recent animal studies, more-realistic exercise protocols have been utilized and results have tended to be less dramatic although supportive of the early findings. Many studies have analyzed the effects of exercise on the development of mammary tumors in rodents using the chemical carcinogens 1-methyl-1-nitrosurea (MNU, a direct-acting carcinogen) and 7,12-dimethyl-benz(a)anthracene (DMBA, a procarcinogen that needs to be activated via metabolism). During the initiation phase (i.e., the first 7 days after carcinogen administration, when the drug undergoes metabolism and alters cells), low levels of treadmill exercise have been shown to reduce DMBA (but not MNU) cancer incidence modestly. In contrast, higher levels of moderate exercise have been shown to inhibit cancer incidence significantly.[63] The data suggest that exercise may affect DMBA metabolism, and not necessarily the response of the mammary gland to carcinogen exposure.[63] Studies analyzing the effects of exercise on the progression phase (i.e., beginning 7 days after administration of the carcinogen and continuing until tumor take) have been less consistent. Thompson's group has found that low-intensity, short-duration exercise actually enhanced the rate of mammary tumor occurrence, whereas at higher moderate intensities of effort, a dose-dependent protective effect was observed.[63] In contrast, Cohen (1991) found a bimodal response, i.e., that low and high intensity enhanced, whereas moderate intensity inhibited, MNU mammary carcinogenesis.[64] Adrianopoulos et al. (1987) found that access to running wheels decreased the induction of colon tumors in response to 1,2 dimethylhydrazine administration.[65]

Several investigators have examined the effect of exercise on the growth and development of transplantable tumors. Welsch et al. (1995) found that growth of transplanted human breast carcinomas in athymic mice was significantly inversely related (r = 0.44) to the mean distance run voluntary per day.[66] Uhlenbruck and Order (1991) found that the growth of a fibrosarcoma was inhibited by treadmill running when the activity was performed before and after transplantation.[67] In contrast, Woods et al. (1994a) demonstrated that moderate or exhaustive treadmill exercise, when performed during (but not before) implantation, did not significantly alter the incidence or growth of a syngeneic mammary adenocarcinoma over a 2-week period.[68] Unfortunately, the protocol may have limited the ability to detect an exercise effect due to the large tumor dose and the short duration of follow-up. In this study, exercise did increase the functional activity of intra-tumoral macrophages.

In addition to modifying the incidence and growth rate of primary tumors, exercise may affect the spread of tumors. Voluntary wheel running activity reduced the number of pulmonary metastases after intravenous injection of CIRAS 1 tumor cells, an effect present only when the animals were allowed access to the wheels for 9 weeks prior to injection.[69] In a follow-up study using the same exercise protocol, MacNeil and Hoffman-Goetz (1993) found that the initial retention of tumor cells was reduced in the wheel-conditioned animals, suggesting that exercise may have reduced the adhesion of tumor cells to the pulmonary vasculature.[70] This same group failed to demonstrate an exercise effect when a more aggressive (i.e., CIRAS 3) tumor was used or a low dose of tumor cells was injected.[71, 72] Others have demonstrated increased tumor retention in the lungs after swimming stress.[73]

Differences in findings are likely related to the variations in exercise protocols (i.e., different intensities, durations, modes of exercise, voluntary vs. forced), cancer-inducing agents (i.e., procarcinogen vs. direct carcinogen) or tumor models, timing of cancer or carcinogen exposure relative to exercise, strains of rodents, and/or confounders such as exercise-induced alterations in body composition and diet. However, the animal evidence certainly suggests that exercise can increase resistance to experimental tumors. In contrast, other psycho-physical stressors (i.e., footshock, restraint, rotation) commonly result in increased tumor incidence and growth.[74] Clearly, there is a need for mechanistic animal studies to determine how exercise promotes this effect.

8.4.2 Effects of Exercise on Anti-Tumor Immune Defenses

Exercise/physical activity may contribute to a reduction in site-specific cancers by different physiological mechanisms. Some purported mechanisms include decreased lifetime exposure to estrogen or other hormones, reduced body fat, enhanced gut motility, improved endogenous antioxidant defenses in the face of increased exercise-induced free-radical formation, and stimulation of anti-tumor immune defenses.[22, 24] Unfortunately, most animal studies have failed to account for plausible biological mechanisms as to how exercise might influence cancer incidence and progression. One way may be through exercise-induced alterations in anti-tumor immune defenses. Indeed, it is well known that both acute and chronic exercise can affect cells of the immune system.[75] However, what is generally not known is whether exercise-induced changes in immune function are related to altered disease susceptibility.

The effects of acute exercise and exercise training on *in vitro* serum immunoglobulin (Ig) synthesis are equivocal.[76] Likewise, small or no differences in baseline Ig concentrations have been reported after either acute exercise or exercise training.[76, 77] However, gross levels of Ig in blood and tissue are not likely to give valuable information relative to the host's ability to mount an antigen-specific antibody response to tumor-specific antigens. Several studies, none of them tumor-derived, have examined the effect of exercise on the production of antibodies to defined antigens. In two human studies,[78, 79] acute, intense exercise did not have an effect on the subsequent generation of antibodies against diphtheria, tetanus, and pneumococcal antigens. In contrast, several studies in rodents have found increased serum antibodies in response to inoculation with diphtheria toxoid,[80] salmonella typhimurium,[81] and keyhole limpet hemocyanin[82] in response to exercise training. This raises the possibility that the chronic exercise might enhance the generation of specific antibodies in response to pathogenic challenge.

Acute and chronic exercise has repeatedly been found to be a potent modulator of NK cell number and function. Of all lymphocyte subsets, NK cells are most responsive to exercise stress. It is typical for NK cell number in peripheral blood to increase 150%–300% immediately following short-term (<60 min), high-intensity exercise, and contribute substantially to the overall lymphocytosis.[75, 83] In addition to NK cell number, NK cell activity (as measured by the *in vitro* lysis of tumor cells) is increased by 40%–100% before falling 25%–40% below pre-exercise levels by 1-h and 2-h of recovery.[75, 83] While most researchers agree that the immediate post-exercise increase in NKCA is due to the recruitment of NK cells into the circulation, they tend to disagree on the reasons for the transient NKCA decrease during recovery.

Although not entirely consistent,[84] several cross-sectional studies support the finding of enhanced NKCA in athletes when compared with non-athletes, in both younger and older groups.[85, 86] Animal data have systematically shown that NKCA is elevated in trained vs. untrained mice and rats.[69, 87] Several studies utilizing moderate endurance training regimens over 8–15 weeks, however, have reported no significant elevation in NKCA among trained vs. untrained humans.[88, 89] Together, these data imply that endurance exercise may have to be intensive and prolonged (i.e., at athletic levels) before NKCA is chronically elevated in humans. Before general conclusions regarding whether exercise improves NK cell tumor defense *in vivo* can be made, important unresolved issues involving destination sites for NK cell trafficking activity need to be addressed —do blood compartment NK cells reflect the NK cell killing capacity of other lymphoid sites, and does exercise affect the ability of NK cells to become further activated by cytokines like IL-2?

Cytolytic T lymphocytes (CTLs) are clearly important in specific anti-cancer defense.[6] Preliminary work suggests that these cells may be susceptible to exercise-induced modulation.[90] Unfortunately, no work has been performed regarding the effects of exercise on the generation of tumor specific CTLs. In addition, other than our study that demonstrated that moderate exercise increased the number and function of intra-tumoral macrophages,[68] no reports exist regarding the effects of exercise on immune function at the tumor-host interface. This is unfortunate, because immune cells in direct association with tumor cells are intimately involved in tumor regulation *in vivo*.

We have shown that both moderate and exhaustive treadmill running over periods of 3–7 d increases the anti-tumor activity of inflammatory and *Propionibacterium acnes- (P. acnes)* activated murine peritoneal Mφs.[91, 92] These effects were not due to altered numbers of Mφs in the assay system but were attributable, in part, to increased production of TNF-γ from TG-elicited Mφs and increased NO production from *P. acnes*-activated Mφs. Likewise, Lotzerich et al. (1990) found that the cytostatic, but not antibody-dependent cytolytic, activity of murine peritoneal Mφs was enhanced after a single exhaustive running session.[93] The role these exercise-induced changes in Mφs anti-tumor activity plays in affecting tumor incidence and progression *in vivo* is unclear. Despite an exercise-induced increase in intra-tumoral Mφ number and activity, Woods et al. (1994) found no changes in tumor incidence or progression.[68] However, exercise was performed during (not prior to) tumorigenesis. In addition, the short duration of the study, the large number of tumor cells transplanted, and the weakly immunogenic nature of the tumor may all have contributed to the lack of an effect. Indeed, recent research using an experimental tumor metastasis model in mice shows that the number of lung tumor metastases resulting from an intravenous injection of B16 melanoma cells was decreased after an acute bout of treadmill exercise. This was associated with an enhancement of anti-tumor cytotoxicity by alveolar Mφs.[94] In response to 4 months of exercise training, resident peritoneal Mφs from young and old mice demonstrated an increased ability to lyse tumor cells *in vitro* when stimulated with IFN-γ and LPS, an effect partly mediated by increased nitric oxide production.[95] Therefore, while the evidence is sparse, there is reason to believe that exercise may beneficially affect anti-tumor immune defense. The big question is, "Do exercise-induced changes in immune function translate into lower incidence rates of specific cancers?" The answer to this question will require further study.

8.4.3 Animal Studies Regarding Diet and Cancer Incidence and Progression

Animal studies involving diet allow the manipulation of individual dietary factors and the determination of their significance on experimental cancer incidence and progression. Dietary issues that have been studied in animal colon-cancer models are unresolved but include the concept of the effects of total fat compared with energy intake, linoleic acid requirements, and interactions of fat with other nutrients.[96] Total dietary fat is generally thought to affect colon tumorigenesis, but there does not appear to be any specific fatty acid that promotes the development of colon cancer. Several studies indicate that n-3 fatty acids from fish sources alter a variety of biological intermediates and inhibit colonic tumorigenesis. Although there are multiple cellular changes elicited by certain fatty acids, including alterations in immune defenses, the current knowledge in this area suggests that specific fatty acid metabolites or their targets are important. Studies examining the role of dietary fiber as an inhibitor of colon cancer in animal models appear to have provided some conflicting results, due mostly to differences in the nature and amount of carcinogen used to induce colon tumors, variation in the composition of the experimental diets, and relative difference in food intake by animals, to cite a few of the methodological problems.[97] However, overall, the feeding of wheat bran appears to inhibit colon tumor development to a greater degree than do other dietary sources of fiber, probably due to decreased gut-transit time or detoxification of cancer-promoting substances in feces.

Increasing dietary fat content increases mammary gland tumorigenesis in laboratory rodents.[98] The effect can be attributed only in part to increasing energy intake, which itself increases tumorigenesis. In addition, restriction of dietary or energy intake without malnutrition, but sufficient to reduce body weight, also reduces mammary gland tumorigenesis. Tumorigenesis in other organs responds similarly to increased fat or decreased energy intake, indicating that the mechanisms are not, or not entirely, specific for the mammary gland. Extrapolations of results between species must always be made with caution, but the marked effects of dietary fat and energy in rodent tumorigenesis models and the findings of human epidemiological studies must be considered in designing diet advice for human breast-cancer prevention. Variations in other dietary factors, such as protein, vitamins, or minerals, above the levels required for normal maintenance seem to have little influence on the genesis or growth of tumors.[99]

8.4.4 Effects of Diet on Anti-Tumor Immune Defenses

The purported mechanisms whereby diet affects cancer incidence and progression are numerous. Examples include the effects of fiber on gut-transit time and bile-acid secretion, the role of dietary antioxidants on protection from free radical damage, and the role of high fat diets on obesity and hormone-dependent cancers. Nutrients enhance or depress immune function depending on type of nutrient and level of its intake. Indeed, it has long been known that malnutrition, especially of protein intake or vitamin A, results in increased susceptibility to infection and lowered immune responses.[100] In contrast, caloric restriction without malnutrition of important macro- and micronutrients can actually increase longevity, reduce cancer incidence, and improve immune function in older animals.[62]

Much recent work has focused on the role of specific dietary factors in influencing immune function. Like information on the role of exercise in modulating anti-tumor immune defense, data is just beginning to accumulate and little is known about whether dietary-induced changes in immune function translate into altered cancer incidence or progression. While it appears that high levels of n-3 polyunsaturated fatty acids (PUFAs) and low levels of n-6 PUFAs seem to be related to lower cancer incidence, the role of these dietary fats on immune function is controversial. On the one hand, diets high in n-3 fats have been shown to decrease mitogen-stimulated lymphocyte proliferation, NK activity, and IL-1, IL-2 and TNF-α production.[101] In contrast, others have performed experiments where n-3 fatty acids were found to be immuno-stimulatory.[102] These differing results may likely be due to the use of different species or the length of dietary manipulation. Clearly, more study is needed in this area.

Vitamin E has been shown to have immunostimulatory effects in a variety of species when administered in quantities in excess of established dietary requirements.[103] Likewise, deficiencies of vitamin E can cause suppression of the immune response system, particularly cell-mediated mechanisms.[103] In animal studies, supplementation with vitamin E protects against infection and is linked to stimulatory effects on the immune system.[103]

Other micronutrients also have diverse immune consequences. For example, deficiency of pyridoxine induces atrophy of lymphoid organs and marked reduction in lymphocyte numbers, impairment of antibody responses and IL-2 production.[104] Dietary copper is important in the prevention of infection in some animal species and T-cell function is defective under deficiency states due to an inability to produce IL-2.[104] Selenium has been linked to viral infection, enhanced T-cell functions and TNF-β induced increase in natural killer cell activity.[104] Beta-carotene increased the number of IL-2R+ T lymphocytes and CD4+ lymphocytes in patients with colon cancer,[105]and has been shown to increase NK cell activity in elderly men.[106] Understanding the molecular and cellular immunological mechanisms involved in nutrient–immune interactions will increase applications for nutrition of the immune system in health and disease.

8.4.5 Experimental Diet and Exercise Combination Studies

Few studies have combined diet and exercise and examined their influence on cancer incidence and progression, and only one study has simultaneously examined anti-tumor immune defense. In one early study, Thompson et al. (1989) found that moderate-intensity treadmill exercise for a short duration could actually stimulate mammary tumorigenesis induced by 7,12-dimethylbenz(a)anthracene (DMBA) in rats fed low- or high-fat diets.[107] This effect predominated in animals fed corn rather than a palm- and corn-oil mixture. In contrast, Cohen et al. (1988) found that voluntary exercise reduced tumor yields and delayed tumor onset in response to N-nitrosomethylurea administration in rats fed high-fat diets.[108] In another study in mice, voluntary exercise had no influence on DMBA-induced cancer in animals fed a standard diet, but decreased tumor incidence under conditions of dietary restriction or high-fat intake.[109] In yet another model, Kazakoff et al. (1996) found that voluntary exercise did not influence cancer burden in hamsters fed high-fat diets and treated with the pancreatic cancer promotor N-nitrosobis-(2-oxopropyl) amine.[110] Dietary L-glutamine supplementation reduced tumor Morris hepatoma 7777 growth, but exercise and glutamine did not act synergistically.[111] Interestingly, glutamine supplementation increased lymphocyte mitogenic proliferation and NK cell numbers in spleen in this same study. These conflicting data are likely the result of different tumor-inducing protocols, experimental species, exercise protocols, and influences of exercise on body composition and food intake. At present, the interaction among exercise, diet, and cancer incidence remains unknown.

8.5 SUMMARY

One way in which exercise and dietary factors might affect all-site cancer incidence and progression is through alteration of anti-cancer immune defenses. Preliminary data have tended to support the hypothesis that moderate exercise may improve immune function, whereas heavy, intense exercise possibly results in immunosuppression.[112] Likewise, many studies have shown that supplementation of certain nutrients or the administration of specific diets can promote or inhibit tumors and enhance or suppress selected anti-tumor immune defenses. The major problem with most studies to date has been the failure to show that exercise- or diet-induced changes in immune function translate into alterations in cancer incidence or progression. Much more research is needed to determine whether the independent or combined effects of proper diet and exercise on cancer prevention are mediated through alterations in anti-tumor immune defenses.

REFERENCES

1. *National Cancer Institute Fact Book*, Bethesda, MD: National Institutes of Health, 1996.
2. Winther, J.F., L. Dreyer, K. Overvad, A. Tjonneland, M., and Gerhardsson de Verdier, Avoidable cancer in the Nordic countries: Diet, obesity, and low physical activity, *APMIS*, 76, 100, 1997.
3. Penn, I., Tumors of the immunocompromised patient, *Annu. Rev. Med.* 39, 63, 1988.
4. Collins, J.L., P.Q. Patek, and M. Cohn, *In vivo* surveillance of tumorigenic cells transformed *in vitro*, *Nature* 299, 169, 1982.
5. Hewitt, H.B, The choice of animal tumors for experimental studies on cancer therapy, *Adv. Cancer Res.* 27, 149, 1978.

6. Schreiber, H., Tumor immunology, in *Fundamental Immunology*, W.E. Paul, Ed., Raven Press, New York, pp. 1143–1178, 1993.

7. Goodman, G.E., I. Hellstrom, and C. Nicaise, Phase I trial of murine monoclonalantibody L6 in breast, colon, ovarian, and lung cancer, *J. Clin. Oncol.* 8, 1083, 1990.

8. Brown, J.P., J.M. Klitzman, I. Hellstrom, R.C. Nowinski, K.E. Hellstrom, Antibody response of mice to chemically induced tumors, *Proc. Natl. Acad. Sci USA* 75, 955, 1978.

9. Old, L.J., Cancer Immunology: the search for specificity, *Cancer Res.* 41, 361, 1981.

10. Alexandroff, A.B., R.A. Robins, A. Murray, K. James, Tumor immunology: false hopes — new horizons? *Immunol. Today* 19, 247, 1998.

11. Herberman, R.B., Natural killer (NK) cells and their possible roles in resistance against disease. *Clin. Immunol. Rev.* 1, 1, 1981.

12. Whiteside, T.L., J. Bryant, R. Day, R. B. Herberman, Natural killer cytotoxicity in the diagnosis of immune dysfunction: Criteria for a reproducible assay, *J. Clin. Lab. Anal.* 4, 102, 1990.

13. Rosenberg, S.A., B.S. Packard, P.M. Aebersold, S.L. Topalian, S.T. Toy, M.T. Lotze, C.A. Seipp, C. Simpson, C. Carter, S., Bock, D. Schwarzentruber, J.P. Wei, D.E. White, Use of tumor-infiltrating lymphocytes and interleukin-2 in the immunotherapy of patients with metastatic melanoma. A preliminary report, *N. Eng. J. Med.* 319, 1676, 1988.

14. Adams, D.O., R. Snyderman, Do macrophages destroy nascent tumors? *J. Natl. Cancer Inst.* 62, 1341, 1979.

15. Whitworth, P.W., C.C. Pak, J. Esgro, E.S. Kleinerman, I.J. Fidler, Macrophages and cancer, *Cancer Metastatsis Rev.* 4, 3139, 1990.

16. El-Bayoumy, K., F.L. Chung, J. Richie, B.S. Reddy, L. Cohen., J. Weisburger, E.L. Wynder, Dietary control of cancer, *Proc. Soc. Exptl. Biol. Med.* 216, 211, 1997.

17. Friedenreich, C.M., T.E. Rohan, A review of physical activity and breast cancer, *Epidemiology* 6, 311, 1995.

18. Hoffman-Goetz, L. and J. Husted, Exercise and cancer: Do the biology and epidemiology correspond? *Exerc. Immunol. Rev.* 1, 81, 1995.

19. Kramer, M.M., C.L. Wells, Does physical activity reduce risk of estrogen-dependent cancer in women? *Med. Sci. Spt. Exerc.* 28, 322, 1996.

20. Oliveria, S.A., I.M. Lee, Is exercise beneficial in the prevention of prostate cancer? *Sport Med.* 23, 271, 1997.

21. Rose, D.P., Dietary fatty acids and prevention of hormone-responsive cancer, *Proc. Soc. Exptl. Biol. Med.* 216, 224, 1997.

22. Shephard, R.J., P.N. Shek, Cancer, immune function, and physical activity. *Can. J. Appl. Physiol.* 20, 1, 1995.

23. Sternfeld, B., Cancer and the protective effect of physical activity: the epidemiological evidence, *Med. Sci. Spt. Exerc.* 24, 1195, 1992.

24. Woods, J.A., Exercise and resistance to neoplasia, *Can. J. Physiol. Pharmacol.* 76, 581, 1998.

25. Albanes, D., A. Blair, P.R. Taylor, Physical activity and risk of cancer in the NHANES I population, *Am. J. Public Health* 79, 744, 1989.

26. Paffenbarger, R.S. Jr., R.T. Hyde, A.L. Wing, Physical activity and incidence of cancer in diverse populations: a preliminary report, *Am. J. Clin. Nutr.* 45, 312, 1987.

27. Whittemore, A.S., J.S. Jr. Paffenbarger, K. Anderson, J.E. Lee, Early precursors of site-specific cancers in college men and women, *J. Nat. Cancer Inst.* 82, 915, 1985.

28. Brownson, R.C., S.H. Zahm, J.C. Chang, A. Blair, Occupational risk of colon cancer, *Am. J. Epidemiol.* 130, 675, 1989.

29. Fredriksson, M., N.O. Bengtsson, L. Hardell, O. Axelson, Colon cancer, physical activity, and occupational exposures, A case-control study. *Cancer* 63, 1838, 1989.
30. Garabrant, D.H., J.M. Peters, T.M. Mack, and I. Bernstein, Job activity and colon cancer risk, *Am. J. Epidemiol.* 119, 1005, 1984.
31. Gerhardsson, M.S., S.E. Norrell, H. Kiviranta, N.L. Pedersson, and A. Ahlbom, Sedentary jobs and colon cancer, *Am. J. Epidemiol.* 123, 775, 1986.
32. Markowitz, S., A. Morabia, K. Garibaldi, and E. Wynder, Effect of occupational and recreational activity on the risk of colorectal cancer among males: A case-control study, *Int. J. Epidemiol.* 21, 1057, 1992.
33. Peters, R.K., D.H. Garabrant, M.C. Yu, and T.M. Mack, A case-control study of occupational and dietary factors in colorectal cancer in young men by subsite, *Cancer Res.* 49, 5459, 1989.
34. Vena, J.E., S. Graham, M. Zielezny, J. Brassure, and M.K. Swanson, Occupational exercise and risk of cancer, *Am. J. Clin. Nutr.* 45, 318, 1987.
35. Enger, S.M., M.P. Longnecker, E.R. Lee, H.D. Frankl, and R.W. Haile, Recent and past physical activity and prevalence of colorectal adenomas, *Br. J. Cancer* 75, 740, 1997.
36. Lee, I.M., R.S. Paffenbarger, Jr., and C.C. Hsieh, Physical activity and risk of developing colorectal cancer among college alumni, *J. Natl. Cancer Inst.* 83, 1324, 1991.
37. Wu, A.H., R.K.R. Paganini-Hill, R.K. Ross, and B.E. Henderson, Alcohol, physical activity, and other risk factors for colorectal cancer: A prospective study, *Br. J. Cancer* 55, 687, 1987.
38. Bernstein, L., B.E. Henderson, R. Hanisch, J. Sullivan-Halley, and R.K. Ross, Physical exercise and reduced risk of breast cancer in young women, *J. Nat. Cancer. Inst.* 86, 1403, 1994.
39. Thune, I., T. Brenn, E. Lund, and M. Gaard, Physical activity and the risk of breast cancer, *N. Eng. J. Med.* 336, 1269, 1997.
40. Zheng, W., S. Shu, J.K. McLaughlin, W.H. Chow, Y.T. Gao, and W.J. Blot, Occupational physical activity and the incidence of cancer of the breast, corpus uteri, and ovary in Shanghai, *Cancer* 71, 3620, 1993.
41. Olson, S.H., J.E. Vena, J.P. Dorn, J.R. Marshall, M. Zielezny,and R. Laughlin, S. Graham, Exercise, occupational activity, and risk of endometrial cancer, *Ann. Epidemiol.* 7, 46, 1997.
42. Lee, I.M., R.S. Paffenbarger, Jr., and C.C. Hsieh, Physical activity and risk of prostatic cancer among college alumni, *Am. J. Epidemiol.* 135, 169, 1992.
43. Frisch, R.E., G. Wyshak, N.L. Albright, T.E. Albright, and I. Schiff, Lower prevalence of non-reproductive system cancers among female former college athletes, *Med. Sci. Spt. Exerc.* 21, 250, 1989.
44. Brownson, R.C., J.C. Chang, J.R. Davis, and C.A. Smith, Physical activity on the job and cancer in Missouri, *Am. J. Public Health* 81, 639, 1991.
45. Severson, R.K., A.M.Y. Nomura, J.S. Grove, and G.N. Stemmermann, A prospective analysis of physical activity and cancer, *Am. J. Epidemiol.* 130, 522, 1989.
46. Giovannucci, E. and W.C. Willet, Dietary factors and risk of colon cancer, *Ann. Med.* 26, 443, 1994.
47. Caygill, C.P., A. Charlett, and M.J. Hill, Fat, fish oil and cancer, *Br. J. Cancer* 74,159, 1996.
48. Howe, G.R., E. Benito, R. Castelleto, J. Cornee, J. Esteve, R.P. Gallagher, J.M. Iscovich, J. Deng-ao, R. Kaaks, and G.A. Kune, Dietary intake of fiber and decreased risk of cancers of the colon and rectum: Evidence from the combined analysis of 13 case-control studies, *J. Natl. Cancer Inst.* 84, 1887, 1992.

49. Wynder, E.L., D.P. Rose, and L.A. Cohen, Diet and breast cancer in causation and therapy, *Cancer* 58, 1804, 1986.

50 Hunter, D.J., D. Spiegelman, H.O. Adami, L. Beeson, I. Van Den Brandt, R. Folsom, G.E. Fraser, R.A. Goldblom, S. Graham, and G.R. Howe, Cohort studies of fat intake and the risk of breast cancer — a pooled analysis, *N. Engl. J. Med.* 334, 356, 1996.

51. Zevernberger, J.L., P.M. Verschuren, and J. Zalalberg, Effect of the amount of dietary fat on the development of mammary tumors in BALB/C-MTV mice, *Cancer* 17, 9, 1992.

52. Merrill, A.H., A.T. Foltz, and D.B. McCormick, Vitamins and cancer, in *Human Nutrition a Comprehensive Treatise. Cancer and Nutrition,* R.B. Alfin-Slater and D. Kritchevsky, Eds., Plenum Press, New York, pp. 262–303, 1991.

53. Birt, D.F. and E. Bresnick, Chemoprevention by nonnutrient components of vegetables and fruits, in *Human Nutrition a Comprehensive Treatise. Cancer and Nutrition* R.B. Alfin-Slater and D. Kritchevsky, Eds., Plenum Press, New York, pp. 221–252, 1991.

54. Graham, S., W. Schotz, and P. Martino, Alimentary factors in the epidemiology of gastric cancer. *Cancer* 30, 927, 1972.

55. Hoffman, S.A., K.E. Paschkis, D.A. DeBias, A. Cantarow, and T.L. Williams, The influence of exercise on the growth of transplanted rat tumors, *Cancer Res.* 22, 597, 1962.

56. Rusch, H.P. and B.E. Kline, The effect of exercise on the growth of a mouse tumor, *Cancer Res.* 4, 116, 1944.

57. Good, R.A. and G. Fernandes, Enhancement of immunologic function and resistance to tumor growth in Balb/c mice by exercise, *Fed. Proceed.* 10, 1040, 1981.

58. Moore, C. and P. Tittle, Muscular activity, body fat, and induced rat mammary tumors, *Surgery* 73, 329, 1973.

59. Rashkis, H.A., Systemic stress as an inhibitor of experimental tumors in Swiss mice, *Science* 116, 169, 1952.

60. Pariza, M.W. and R.K. Boutwell, Historical perspective: Calories and energy expenditure in carcinogenesis, *Am. J. Clin. Nutr.* 45, 151, 1987.

61. Volk, M.J., T.D. Pugh, M. Kim, C.H. Frith, R.A. Daynes, W.B. Ershler, W.B., and R. Weindruch, Dietary restriction from middle age attenuates age-associated lymphoma development and interleukin-6 dysregulation in C57BL/6 mice, *Cancer Res.* 54, 3054, 1994.

62. Weindruch, R., Immunogerontologic outcomes of dietary restriction started in adulthood, *Nutrition Rev.* 53, S66, 1995.

63. Thompson, H.J., Effect of exercise intensity and duration on the induction of mammary carcinogenesis, *Cancer Res.* 54, 1960s, 1994.

64. Cohen, L.A., Physical activity and cancer, *Cancer Prevention* 26, 1, 1991.

65. Adrianopoulos, G., R.L. Nelson, C.T. Bombeck, and G. Souza, The influence of physical activity in 1,2 dimethylhydrazine induced colon carcinogenesis in the rat, *Anticancer Res.* 7, 849, 1987.

66. Welsch, M.A., L.A. Cohen, and C.W. Welsch, Inhibition of growth of human breast carcinoma xenografts by energy expenditure via voluntary exercise in athymic mice fed a high-fat diet, *Nutr. Cancer* 23, 309, 1995.

67. Uhlenbruck, G. and U. Order, Can endurance sports stimulate immune mechanisms against cancer and metastasis? *Int. J. Spt. Med.* 12, S53, 1991.
68. Woods, J.A., J.M. Davis, M.L. Kohut, A. Ghaffar, E.P. Mayer, and R.R. Pate, Effects of exercise on the immune response to cancer, *Med. Sci. Spt. Exerc.* 26, 1109, 1994.
69. MacNeil, B. and L. Hoffman-Goetz, Exercise training and tumour metastasis in mice: Influence of time of exercise and onset, *Anticancer Res.* 13, 2085, 1993.
70. MacNeil, B. and L. Hoffman-Goetz, Chronic exercise enhances *in vivo* and *in vitro* cytotoxic mechanisms of natural immunity in mice, *J. Appl. Physiol.* 74, 388, 1993.
71. Hoffman-Goetz, L., B. MacNeil, A. Arumugum, and J.R. Simpson, Differential effects of exercise and housing condition on murine natural killer cell activity and tumor growth, *Int. J. Spt. Med.* 2, 167, 1992.
72. Jadeski, L. and L. Hoffman-Goetz. Exercise and *in vivo* natural cytotoxicity against tumour cells of varying metastatic capacity, *Clin. Expt. Metastasis* 14, 138, 1996.
73. Ben-Eliyahu, S., R. Yirmiya, Y. Shavit, and J.C. Liebeskind, Stress increases metastatic spread of a mammary tumor in rats: evidence for mediation by the immune system, *Brain, Behav. Immun.* 5, 193, 1991.
74. Riley, V., Psychoneuroendocrine influences on immunocompetence and neoplasia, *Science* 212, 1100, 1981.
75. Shephard, R.J., Physical activity, training and the immune response, Cooper Publishing, Carmel, IN, 1997.
76. Mackinnon, L.T., Immunoglobulin, antibody, and exercise, *Exerc. Immunol. Rev.* 2, 1, 1996.
77. Nehlsen-Cannerella, S.L., D.C. Nieman, J. Jessen, L. Chang, G. Gusewitch, G.G. Blix, and E. Ashley, The effects of acute moderate exercise on lymphocyte function and serum immunoglobulin levels, *Int. J. Spt. Med.* 12, 391, 1991.
78. Bruunsgaard, H., A. Hartkopp, T. Mohr, H.. Konradsen, I. Heron, C.H. Mordhorst, and B.K. Pedersen, In vivo cell-mediated immunity and vaccination response following prolonged, intense exercise, *Med. Sci. Spt. Exerc.* 29, 1176, 1997.
79. Eskola, J., O. Ruuskanen, and E. Soppi, Effect of sport stress on lymphocyte transformation and antibody formation, *Clin. Expt. Immunol.* 32, 339, 1978.
80. Douglass J.H., The effects of physical tracing on the immunological response in mice, *J. Sports Med. Phys. Fitness* 14, 48, 1974.
81. Liu Y.G. and S.Y. Wang, The enhancing effect of exercise on the production of antibody to Salmonella typhi in mice, *Immunol. Lett.* 14, 117, 1987.
82. Kaufman J.C., T.J. Harris, J. Higgins and A.S. Maisel, Exercise-induced enhancement of immune function in the rat, *Circulation*, 90, 525, 1994.
83. Pedersen, B.K. and H. Ullum, NK cell response to physical activity: possible mechanisms of action, *Med. Sci. Spt. Exerc.* 26,140, 1994.
84. Shinkai, S., H. Kohno, K. Kimura, T. Komura, H. Asai, R. Inai, K. Oka, Y. Kurokawa, and R.J. Shephard, Physical activity and immune senescence in men, *Med. Sci. Sports Exerc.* 27, 1516, 1995.
85. Nieman, D.C., K.S. Buckley, D.A. Henson, B.J. Warren, J. Suttles, J.C. Ahle, S. Simandle. O.R. Fagoaga, and S.L. Nehlsen-Cannarella. Immune function in marathon runners vs. sedentary controls. *Med. Sci. Sports Exerc.* 27, 986, 1995.

86. Pedersen, B.K., N. Tvede, L.D. Christensen, K. Klarlund, S. Kragbak, and J. Halkjr-Kristensen, Natural killer cell activity in peripheral blood of highly trained and untrained persons, *Int. J. Sports Med.* 10,129, 1989.

87. Jonsdottir, I.H., A. Asea, and P. Hoffman, Voluntary chronic exercise augments in vivo natural immunity in rats, *J. Appl. Physiol.* 80, 1799, 1995.

88. Nieman, D.C., S.L. Nehlsen-Cannarella, P.A. Markoff, A.J. Balk-Lamberton, H. Yang, D.B. Chritton, J.W. Lee, and K. Arabatzis, The effects of moderate exercise training on natural killer cells and acute upper respiratory tract infections, *Int. J. Sports Med.* 11, 467, 1990.

89. Nieman, D.C., D.A. Henson, G. Gusewitch, B.J. Warren, R.C. Dotson, D.E. Butterworth, and S.L. Nehlsen-Cannarella, Physical activity and immune function in elderly women, *Med. Sci. Sports Exercise* 25, 823, 1993.

90. Wolters, B.W., M.A. Ceddia, C.A. Germann, and J.A. Woods, Exhaustive exercise increases cytotoxic T lymphocyte anti-EL-4 tumor immunity, *Med. Sci. Spt. Exerc.* 29, S158, 1997.

91. Woods, J.A., J.M. Davis, E.P. Mayer, A. Ghaffar, and R.R. Pate, Exercise increases inflammatory macrophage anti-tumor cytotoxicity, *J. Appl. Physiol.* 75, 879, 1993.

92. Woods, J.A., J.M. Davis, E.P. Mayer, A. Ghaffar, and R.R. Pate, Effects of exercise on macrophage activation for anti-tumor cytotoxicity, *J. Appl. Physiol.* 76, 2177, 1994.

93. Lotzerich, H., H.G. Fehr, and H. Appell, Potentiation of cytostatic but not cytolytic activity of murine macrophages after running stress, *Int. J. Spt. Med.* 11, 61, 1990.

94. Davis, J.M., M.L. Kohut, D.A. Jackson, L.M. Hertler-Colbert, E.P. Mayer, and A. Ghaffar, Exercise effects on lung tumor metastases and *in vitro* alveolar macrophage anti-tumor cytotoxicity, *Am. J. Physiol.* 274, R1454, 1998.

95. Lu, Q., M.A. Ceddia, E.A. Price, and J.A. Woods, Chronic exercise increases macrophage-mediated anti-tumor cytolytic function in young and old mice, *Am. J. Physiol.* 276, R482, 1999.

96. Klurfeld D.M. and A.W. Bull, Fatty acids and colon cancer in experimental models, *Am. J. Clin. Nutr.* 66, 1530S, 1997.

97. Reddy B.S., Dietary fiber and colon cancer: animal model studies, *Prev. Med.* 16, 559, 1987.

98. Rogers A.E. Diet and breast cancer: studies in laboratory animals. *J. Nutr.* 127, 933S, 1997.

99. Carroll, K.K., Experimental evidence of dietary factors and hormone-dependent cancers, *Cancer Res* 35, 3374, 1975.

100. Chandra, R., Immune response in undernutrition and overnutrition: Basic considerations and applied significance, *Nutrition* 5, 297, 1989.

101. Calder P.C., Fat chance of immunomodulation, *Immunol. Today* 19, 244, 1998.

102. Netea, M.G., B.J. Kullberg, W.L. Blok, and J. Van der Meer, Immunomodulation by n-3 polyunsaturated fatty acids, *Immunol. Today* 120, 103, 1999.

103. Meydani S.N. and A.A. Beharka, Recent developments in vitamin E and immune response, *Nutr. Rev.* 56, S49,1998.

104. Harbige L.S., Nutrition and immunity with emphasis on infection and autoimmune disease, *Nutr. Health* 10, 285, 1996.

105. Kazi N., R. Radvany, T. Oldham, A. Keshavarzian, T.O. Frommel, C. Libertin, and S. Mobarhan, Immunomodulatory effect of beta-carotene on T lymphocyte subsets in patients with resected colonic polyps and cancer, *Nutr. Cancer* 28,140, 1997.

106. Santos M.S., J.M. Gaziano, L.S. Leka, A.A. Beharka, C.H. Hennekens, and S.N. Meydani, Beta-carotene-induced enhancement of natural killer cell activity in elderly men: an investigation of the role of cytokines, *Am. J .Clin. Nutr.* 68,164, 1998.

107. Thompson H.J., A.M. Ronan, K.A. Ritacco, and A.R. Tagliaferro, Effect of type and amount of dietary fat on the enhancement of rat mammary tumorigenesis by exercise, *Cancer Res* 49, 1904, 1989.

108. Cohen L., K.W. Choi, and C.X. Wang, Influence of dietary fat, caloric restriction, and voluntary exercise on N-nitrosomethylurea-induced mammary tumorigenesis in rats, *Cancer Res* 48, 4276, 1988.

109. Lane, H.W., P. Teer, R.E. Keith, M.T. White, and S. Strahan, Reduced energy intake and moderate exercise reduce mammary tumor incidence in virgin female BALB/c mice treated with 7,12- dimethylbenz(a)anthracene, *J. Nutr.* 121, 1883, 1991.

110. Kazakoff K; T. Cardesa, J. Liu, T.E. Adrian, D. Bagchi, M. Bagchi, D.F. Birt, and P.M. Pour, Effects of voluntary physical exercise on high-fat-diet-promoted pancreatic carcinogenesis in the hamster model, *Nutr. Cancer* 26, 265, 1996.

111. Shewchuk L.D., V.E. Baracos, and C. Field, Dietary L-glutamine supplementation reduces the growth of the Morris Hepatoma 7777 in exercise-trained and sedentary rats, *J. Nutr.* 127, 158, 1997.

112. Brines, R., L. Hoffman-Goetz, and B.K. Pedersen, Can you exercise to make your immune system fitter? *Immunol. Today* 17, 252, 1996.

CHAPTER 9

Exercise, Immune Function, and Nutrition: Summary and Future Perspectives

Bente Klarlund Pedersen and David Nieman

CONTENTS

1-8493-0741-4/00/$0.00+$.50

9.1. AN ACUTE BOUT OF EXERCISE

9.1.1   What Is Known?

Research since the 1980s has shown that the response of blood mononuclear cells to a bout of exercise is highly stereotypical. Intense exercise recruits a high number of lymphocytes to the blood compartment, and most of these are natural-killer (NK) and T cells.[1] The increased number of T cells is represented largely by memory CD8+ cells that lack the CD28 surface receptor.[2] This phenotype is typical of cells with a low proliferative capacity, and is consistent with the finding that cells with shortened telomere lengths can be isolated from the blood during exercise.[2] Together, these data suggest that lymphocytes are mobilized during exercise from peripheral compartments such as the spleen, the intestine, and the lymph nodes, and are consistent with an attenuated lymphocytosis during exercise in patients without spleens.[3]

Following intense exercise, the total lymphocyte count in the blood compartment declines. This exercise-induced lymphocytopenia could be due to a redistribution of the lymphocytes to organs (e.g., muscles or lungs), and/or a consequence of apoptosis. When cellular immune function is assessed by *in vitro* measurements, NK- and LAK-cell activity, lymphocyte proliferative responses, and the *in vitro* production of immunoglobulins decline. *In vivo* immune measurements have shown that the delayed type hypersensitivity reaction to recall antigens introduced into the skin is impaired following strenuous exercise, whereas antibody responses following vaccination remain normal.[4] Several reports describe that the concentration and output of IgA in saliva are decreased by exercise.[5]

Exercise is also associated with high plasma levels of several pro- and anti-inflammatory cytokines and chemokines. These include tumor necrosis factor alpha (TNF-α), interleukin (IL)-6, IL-1receptor antagonist (IL-1ra), IL-8, IL-10, TNF-receptors (TNF-R) and macrophage inhibitory proteins (MIP).[6,7,8]

9.1.2   What Is Not Known?

The clinical significance of the exercise-induced immune changes is not known. Although athletes report an increased frequency of upper respiratory tract symptoms after a marathon[9] and animal studies suggest an increased virulence of certain microorganisms when exercise is performed during the incubation period,[10] the link between these findings and altered immunity following heavy exertion has not been established in humans.

The increased concentration of plasma cytokines after strenuous exercise has some similarity to that of trauma and sepsis. One unique difference is the disproportionate increase in plasma levels of IL-6 relative to other pro-inflammatory cytokines following prolonged and intensive exercise. The stimuli for this phenomenon are not yet defined. One hypothesis is that IL-6 is a marker of "suffering cells" in the skeletal muscle, and that IL-6 initiates healing processes.

9.2. CHRONIC EXERCISE AND IMMUNE FUNCTION

9.2.1 What Is Known?

In contrast to the large number of studies on the immune response to acute exercise, much less is known on the effect of physical training on immune function. This is in part due to the difficulties in separating acute and chronic exercise training effects on immunity. Depending on the immune component measured, changes induced by intense physical exercise may last more than 24 hours.[11] The influence of chronic exercise has been studied in both animal and human models, using cross-sectional and longitudinal designs. Cross-sectional studies have shown increased natural immunity in elite cyclists,[12, 13] runners,[14] and highly conditioned elderly subjects,[15] while others have reported no difference between trained and untrained subjects.[16, 17] Most longitudinal studies[15–20] with human subjects have shown no change in NK-cell activity when healthy elderly subjects,[15] patients with rheumatoid arthritis,[18] or obese women[20] were randomized to 8 to 15 weeks of exercise training. In contrast to the human studies, several animal studies using training protocols of varying length and intensity support the findings of increased resting levels of natural cytotoxicity after voluntary exercise.[21–25]

9.2.2 What Is Not Known?

The findings on NK-cell activity and training are controversial, and it is possible that the enhanced activity reported in some groups of athletes may be related to factors other than exercise, such as nutrient intake or the residual effect of the previous day's exercise bout. It is curious that of all the immune cells found in the blood compartment, only the activity of the NK cell has been related to athletic endeavor. The clinical implications are unknown, but long-term benefits may include enhanced immunosurveillance against certain types of viruses and cancer.

9.3. EXERCISE AND IMMUNE FUNCTION — WHY MIGHT NUTRIENT INTAKE PLAY A ROLE?

The mechanisms underlying exercise-associated immune changes are multifactorial and include neuroendocrinological factors such as epinephrine, norepinephrine, growth hormone, cortisol, and beta-endorphin.[26] Altered protein metabolism and decreased plasma glutamine concentrations as a result of muscular activity have been hypothesized to influence lymphocyte function.[27] A decrease in plasma glucose during prolonged and intensive exercise has been related to elevated stress hormone levels and, as a consequence, immune function.[28] Furthermore, free oxygen radicals and prostaglandins (PG) released by activated neutrophils and monocytes during exercise may influence the function of lymphocytes. Thus, nutritional supplementation with glutamine, carbohydrate, antioxidants, or PG-inhibitors has been hypothesized to influence exercise-associated changes in immune function.

9.4. GLUTAMINE HYPOTHESIS

Under intense physical exercise, the demands by muscle and other organs for glutamine may create a deficit to the lymphoid organs, temporarily influencing immunity. Thus, factors that directly or indirectly influence glutamine synthesis or release could theoretically influence the function of lymphocytes and mono-cytes.[29,30]

9.4.1   WHAT IS KNOWN?

Following intense long-term exercise and other physical stress disorders, the plasma concentration of glutamine declines.[31, 32, 33, 34] Glutamine added to cell cultures *in vitro* enhances lymphocyte proliferation and LAK cell activity, but has no effect on NK cell activity.[35] Furthermore, *in vitro* experiments have shown that glutamine stimulates IL-2 and IFN-γ production, without influencing the production of IL-1β, IL-6, or TNF-α.[36] In one study, glutamine added to *in vitro* assays was unable to abolish the post-exercise decline in proliferative responses, and did not normalize low lymphocyte proliferation rates in HIV seropositive patients.[35]

A study by Castell et al.[37] found that glutamine supplementation decreased the incidence of upper respiratory tract infection (URTI) after a marathon. MacKinnon et al.,[38] however, were unable to verify this finding in an overtraining study of elite swimmers. In two recent placebo-controlled studies,[39, 40] glutamine abolished the post-exercise decline in plasma glutamine without influencing post-exercise impairment of NK- and LA-cell function, or mitogen-induced proliferative responses. These studies did not support the hypothesis that the post-exercise decline in immune function is caused by a decrease in plasma glutamine. This interpretation is consistent with the finding that decreased immune function *in vitro* is seen only if the glutamine concentration falls below 10% of physiological concentrations, well below the 60% level found after marathon-type exertion.

9.4.2   FUTURE PERSPECTIVES

A few more glutamine-supplementation studies may be warranted to finally reject the glutamine hypothesis. Future studies should determine if plasma glutamine is lowered in overtraining, as has been suggested by some authors,[41] and whether a link exists between resting levels of plasma glutamine, immune function, and risk of obtaining an infection in large groups of athletes.

9.5 CARBOHYDRATE — HYPOTHESIS

Earlier research had established that a reduction in blood glucose levels is linked to hypothalamic–pituitary–adrenal activation, an increased release of adrenocorticotrophic hormone and cortisol, increased plasma growth hormone, decreased insulin, and a variable effect on blood epinephrine level.[28] Given the link between stress hormones and immune responses to prolonged and intensive exercise,[26] it was hypothesized that carbohydrate ingestion should maintain plasma glucose concentrations, attenuate increases in stress hormones, and thereby diminish changes in immunity.

9.5.1 What Is Known?

This hypothesis has been tested in a number of studies[42–48] using double-blind, placebo-controlled, randomized designs. Carbohydrate beverage ingestion before, during (about 1 l/h), and after 2.5 h of exercise has been associated with higher plasma glucose levels, an attenuated cortisol and growth hormone response, fewer perturbations in blood immune cell counts, lower granulocyte and monocyte phagocytosis and oxidative burst activity, and an increase in plasma IL-6 and IL-1ra. Overall, the hormonal and immune responses to carbohydrate compared with placebo ingestion were diminished. Some immune variables were affected slightly by carbohydrate ingestion (for example, granulocyte and monocyte function), while others were strongly influenced (e.g., plasma cytokine concentrations and blood cell counts).

9.5.2 Future Perspectives

The clinical significance of the carbohydrate-induced effects on the endocrine and immune systems awaits further research. At this point, the data indicate that athletes ingesting carbohydrate beverages before, during, and after prolonged and intensive exercise should experience lowered physiologic stress. Research to determine whether carbohydrate ingestion will improve host protection against viruses in endurance athletes during periods of intensified training or following competitive endurance events is warranted. Also, it needs to be established whether the diminished cytokine response is due to direct or indirect mechanisms. Furthermore, the effect of carbohydrate supplementation on muscle damage should be investigated. It would be of interest to determine if carbohydrate supplementation can alter the acute phase response to clinical stress disorders such as sepsis and trauma, conditions that have some parallels to exercise stress.

9.6 POLYUNSATURATED FATTY ACID HYPOTHESIS

There are two principal classes of polyunsaturated fatty acids (PUFA): the n-6 and the n-3 families.[49] The precursor of the n-6 family is linoleic acid, which is converted to arachidonic acid, the precursor of PG and leukotrienes (LT), which have potent proinflammatory and immunoregulatory properties. The precursor of the n-3 family of PUFA is α-linoleic acid. The n-6/n-3 ratio can be decreased by ingesting a diet rich in n-3 fatty acids, thus potentially negating PGE-2-mediated immunosuppression. Acute exercise induces high levels of PGE-2. Although results have been less than clear regarding the effect of PG inhibitors on post-exercise immune impairment,[50, 51] it has been hypothesized that n-3 PUFA supplementation may alter exercise-induced immune changes by a mechanism that involves PG or alteration of the fluidity and structure of cell membranes.

9.6.1   N-3 PUFA — What is Known?

The possible interaction among intense acute exercise, immune function, and PUFA was examined in inbred female C57Bl/6 mice.[52] The animals received either a natural-ingredient diet or a diet supplemented with various oils such as beef tallow, safflower, fish oil or linseed oil for an 8-week period. In the group receiving 18:3 (n-3) linseed oil, post-exercise immunosuppression (immunoglobulin M plaque-forming cell response) was abolished.

In a study of elderly humans,[53] neutrophil and monocyte function after an *in vivo* inflammatory stress was measured following dietary modification of fatty acids. *In vivo* neutrophil degranulation was assessed by plasma elastase concentrations, and monocyte function was assessed by IL-1β secretion *in vitro*. In response to eccentric exercise, subjects in the placebo group had no apparent elastase response, whereas those taking fish-oil supplements responded with a significant increase (142%) in plasma elastase similar to responses of younger reference subjects. There was no effect of fish oil on IL-1β secretion.

9.6.2   N-3 PUFA — Future Perspectives

Although animal experiments indicate that the cytokine response following endotoxin injection is diminished when animals are pretreated with n-3 PUFA, there are no published studies on the influence of n-3 PUFA-rich diets on exercise-induced increases in pro-inflammatory cytokines. Research in this area is warranted.[54] Also, the combined effect of long-term training and diets rich or poor in n-3 or n-6 PUFAs would be of interest.

9.7. ANTIOXIDANT — HYPOTHESIS

During exercise, the large increase in oxygen utilization is associated with an increased production of reactive oxygen species (as measured through the blood glutathione redox status). In theory, antioxidant supplements may neutralize the reactive oxygen species produced by neutrophils during phagocytosis.[55, 56]

9.7.1   What Is Known?

Peters et al.[57] evaluated the effect of vitamin C on the incidence of URTI during the 2-week period following the 90-km Comrades Ultramarathon. Symptoms of URTI were reported by 68% of runners in the placebo group, significantly more than in the vitamin C supplementation group where only 33% reported URTI symptoms when taking 600 mg vitamin C daily for 3 weeks prior to the race. In another study, Peters et al.[58] found that vitamin A supplementation had an insignificant effect on URTI symptoms in ultramarathoners.

Only one study[59] has evaluated the effect of vitamin C on lymphocyte function and stress hormone levels after exercise. Supplementation with vitamin C did not influence exercise-induced alterations in leukocyte subsets, NK-cell activity, lymphocyte proliferative responses, granulocyte phagocytosis and oxidative burst activity, and catecholamines and cortisol. In a recent double-blind, placebo-controlled study by Nielsen et al.,[60] N-acetylcysteine (6 g daily for 3 days) had no effect on exercise-induced suppression of lymphocyte proliferation or NK-cell activity.

A double-blind, placebo-controlled study investigated the effect of vitamin E supplementation for 48 h on the exercise-induced acute phase response.[61] The volunteers were young (average age 25 years) and elderly (average age 65 years) sedentary men. They performed 45 min of eccentric exercise (downhill treadmill running). Twenty-four hours after a single session of eccentric exercise, endotoxin-induced secretion of IL-1β was augmented in cells obtained from the placebo subjects, but not those from the vitamin E-supplemented subjects.[61] The effect of vitamin E on IL-1β was not apparently related to changes in PGE-2. Oxygen radicals enhance endotoxin-induced IL-1 production.[62] Furthermore, the concentration of these reactants increases with exercise.[63] Thus, the effects of vitamin E on the secretion of IL-1β is consistent with a mechanism involving oxygen radicals.

9.7.2   Future Perspectives

There is a lack of reliable methods to estimate *in vivo* oxidative stress. One possibility would be to include measurement of the so-called iso-prostatanes. There is a need for studies testing varying doses of antioxidant vitamins, because high compared with moderate doses may not always be beneficial.[64] There are few studies available testing the effect of antioxidant vitamins on cellular immune function and plasma cytokines, but much more research in this area is needed before definitive conclusions can be drawn.

9.8 CONCLUSION

Exercise produces an acute-phase response similar to what occurs during physical trauma and sepsis. Of all nutrient components studied heretofore, only carbohydrate supplementation has shown significant effects on exercise-induced immune changes. Although clinical relevance has not been established, supplementation studies may serve to elucidate important mechanisms. For example, it has been hypothesized that post-exercise immune changes are linked to increased infection rates, and that the cytokine response to exercise may be associated with muscle soreness and damage. If nutrient supplementation (especially carbohydrate) has an influence on exercise-induced immunity, infection rates, and muscle soreness, the next logical step is to determine how and why.

REFERENCES

1.   Hoffman-Goetz, L. and Pedersen, B.K., Exercise and the immune system: a model of the stress response?, *Immunol. Today*, 15, 382, 1994.

2. Bruunsgaard, H., Jensen, M.S., Schjerling, P., Halkjaer-Kristensen, J., Ogawa, S., Skinhoj, P., and Pedersen, B.K., Exercise induces recruitment of lymphocytes with an activated phenotype and short telomeres in young and elderly humans, *Life Sci.*, (in press).

3. Nielsen, H.B., Halkjaer-Kristensen, J., Christensen, N.J., and Pedersen, B.K., Splenectomy impairs lymphocytosis during maximal exercise, *Am. J. Physiol.*, 272, R1847, 1997.

4. Bruunsgaard, H., Hartkopp, A., Mohr, T., Konradsen, H., Heron, I., Mordhorst, C.H., and Pedersen, B.K., *In vivo* cell mediated immunity and vaccination response following prolonged intense exercise, *Med. Sci. Sports Exerc.*, 29, 1176, 1997.

5. Mackinnon, L.T., Chick, T.W., van As, A., and Tomasi, T.B., The effect of exercise on secretory and natural immunity, *Adv. Exp. Med. Biol.*, 216A, 869, 1987.

6. Ostrowski, K., Rohde, T., Zacho, M., Asp, S., and Pedersen, B.K., Evidence that IL-6 is produced in skeletal muscle during intense long-term muscle activity, *J. Physiol. (Lond.)*, 508, 949, 1998.

7. Ostrowski, K., Hermann, C., Bangash, A., Schjerling, P., Nielsen, J.N., and Pedersen, B.K., A trauma-like elevation in plasma cytokines in humans in response to treadmill running, *J. Physiol. (Lond.)*, 508, 949, 1998.

8. Ostrowski, K., Rohde, T., Asp, S., Schjerling, P., and Pedersen, B.K., The cytokine balance and strenuous exercise: TNF-alpha, IL-2beta, IL-6, IL-1ra, sTNF-r1, sTNF-r2, and IL-10, *J. Physiol. (Lond.)*, 515, 287, 1999.

9. Nieman, D.C., Exercise, upper respiratory tract infection, and the immune system, *Med. Sci. Sports Exerc.*, 26, 128, 1994.

10. Friman, G. and Ilback, N.G., Exercise and infection — interaction, risks and benefits, *Scand. J. Med. Sci. Sports*, 2, 177, 1992.

11. Pedersen, B.K. and Nieman, D.C., Exercise immunology: Regulation and integration. *Immunol. Today*, 19, 204, 1998.

12. Pedersen, B.K., Tvede, N., Christensen, L.D., Klarlund, K., Kragbak, S., and Halkjr Kristensen, J., Natural killer cell activity in peripheral blood of highly trained and untrained persons, *Int. J. Sports Med.*, 10, 129, 1989.

13. Tvede, N., Steensberg, J., Baslund, B., Halkjaer Kristensen, J., and Pedersen, B.K., Cellular immunity in highly trained elite racing cyclists during periods of training with high and low intensity, *Scand. J. Med. Sci. Sports*, 1, 163, 1991.

14. Nieman, D.C., Buckley, K.S., Henson, D.A., Warren, B.J., Suttles, J., Ahle, J.C., Simandle, S., Fagoaga, O.R., and Nehlsen Cannarella, S.L., Immune function in marathon runners versus sedentary controls, *Med. Sci. Sports Exerc.*, 27, 986, 1995.

15. Nieman, D.C., Henson, D.A., Gusewitch, G., Warren, B.J., Dotson, R.C., Butterworth, D.E., and Nehlsen-Cannarella, S.L., Physical activity and immune function in elderly women, *Med. Sci. Sports Exerc.*, 25, 823, 1993.

16. Brahmi, Z., Thomas, J.E., Park, M., and Dowdeswell, I.R., The effect of acute exercise on natural-killer-cell activity of trained and sedentary human subjects, *J. Clin. Immunol.*, 5, 321, 1985.

17. Nieman, D.C., Brendle, D., Henson, D.A., Suttles, J., Cook, V.D., Warren, B.J., Butterworth, D.E., Fagoaga, O.R., and Nehlsen Cannarella, S.L., Immune function in athletes versus nonathletes, *Int. J. Sports Med.*, 16, 329, 1995.

18. Barnes, C.A., Forster, M.J., Fleshner, M., Ahanotu, E.N., Laudenslager, M.L., Mazzeo, R.S., Maier, S.F. and Lal, H., Exercise does not modify spatial memory, brain autoimmunity, or antibody response in aged F-344 rats, *Neurobiol. Aging*, 12, 47, 1991.

19. Crist, D.M., Mackinnon, L.T., Thompson, R.F., Atterbom, H.A., and Egan, P.A., Physical exercise increases natural cellular-mediated tumor cytotoxity in elderly women, *Gerontology*, 35, 66, 1989.

20. Nieman, D.C., Nehlsen-Cannarella, S.L., Markoff, P.A., Balk Lamberton, A.J., Yang, H., Chritton, D.B., Lee, J.W., and Arabatzis, K., The effects of moderate exercise training on natural killer cells and acute upper respiratory tract infections, *Int. J. Sports Med.*, 11, 467, 1990.

21. Hoffman-Goetz, L., Arumugam, Y., and Sweeny, L., Lymphokine activated killer cell activity following voluntary physical activity in mice, *J. Sports Med. Phys. Fit.*, 34, 83, 1994.

22. Hoffman-Goetz, L., MacNeil, B., Arumugam, Y., and Randall Simpson, J., Differential effects of exercise and housing condition on murine natural killer cell activity and tumor growth, *Int. J. Sports Med.*, 13, 167, 1992.

23. MacNeil, B. and Hoffman-Goetz, L., Chronic exercise enhances *in vivo* and *in vitro* cytotoxic mechanisms of natural immunity in mice, *J. Appl. Physiol.*, 74, 388, 1993.

24. MacNeil, B., and Hoffman-Goetz, L., Effect of exercise on natural cytotoxicity and pulmonary tumor metastases in mice, *Med. Sci. Sports Exerc.*, 25, 922, 1993.

25. MacNeil, B., and Hoffman-Goetz, L., Exercise training and tumor metastasis in mice: influence of time of exercise onset, *Anticancer Res.*, 13, 2085, 1993.

26. Pedersen, B.K., Bruunsgaard, H., Klokker, M., Kappel, M., MacLean, D.A., Nielsen, H.B., Rohde, T., Ullum, H., and Zacho, M., Exercise-induced immunomodulation — possible roles of neuroendocrine factors and metabolic factors, *Int. J. Sports Med.*, 18, S2, 1997.

27. Newsholme, E.A. and Parry Billings, M., Properties of glutamine release from muscle and its importance for the immune system, *J. Parenter. Enteral. Nutr.*, 14, 63S, 1990.

28. Nieman, D.C. and Pedersen, B.K., Exercise and immune function: recent development, *Sports Med.*, 27, 73, 1999.

29. Newsholme, E.A., Biochemical mechanisms to explain immunosuppression in well-trained and overtrained athletes, *Int. J. Sports Med.*, 15, S142, 1994.

30. Newsholme, E.A., Psychoimmunology and cellular nutrition: an alternative hypothesis [editorial], *Biol. Psychiatry*, 27, 1, 1990.

31. Parry Billings, M., Budgett, R., Koutedakis, Y., Blomstrand, E., Brooks, S., Williams, C., Calder, P.C., Pilling, S., Baigrie, R., and Newsholme, E.A., Plasma amino acid concentrations in the overtraining syndrome: possible effects on the immune system, *Med. Sci. Sports Exerc.*, 24, 1353, 1992.

32. Keast, D., Arstein, D., Harper, W., Fry, R.W., and Morton, A.R., Depression of plasma glutamine concentration after exercise stress and its possible influence on the immune system, *Med. J. Aust.*, 162, 15, 1995.

33. Essen, P., Wernerman, J., Sonnenfeld, T., Thunell, S., and Vinnars, E., Free amino acids in plasma and muscle during 24 hours post-operatively — a descriptive study, *Clin. Physiol.*, 12, 163, 1992.

34. Lehmann, M., Huonker, M., Dimeo, F., Heinz, N., Gastmann, U., Treis, N., Steinacker, J.M., Keul, J., Kajewski, R., and Haussinger, D., Serum amino acid concentrations in nine athletes before and after the 1993 Colmar ultra triathlon, *Int. J. Sports Med.*, 16, 155, 1995.

35. Rohde, T., Ullum, H., Palmo, J., Halkjaer Kristensen, J., Newsholme, E.A., and Pedersen, B.K., Effects of glutamine on the immune system-influence of muscular exercise and HIV infection, *J. Appl. Physiol.*, 79, 146, 1995.

36. Rohde, T., MacLean, D.A., and Pedersen, B.K., Glutamine, lymphocyte proliferation and cytokine production, *Scand. J. Immunol.*, (in press).

37. Castell, L.M., Poortmans, J.R., and Newsholme, E.A., Does glutamine have a role in reducing infections in athletes?, *Eur. J. Appl. Physiol.*, 73, 488, 1996.
38. Mackinnon, L.T. and Hooper, S.L., Plasma glutamine and upper respiratory tract infection during intensified training in swimmers, *Med. Sci. Sports Exerc.*, 28, 285, 1996.
39. Rohde, T., MacLean, D., and Pedersen, B.K., Effect of glutamine on changes in the immune system induced by repeated exercise, *Med. Sci. Sports Exerc.*, 30, 856, 1998.
40. Rohde, T., Asp, S., MacLean, D.A., and Pedersen, B.K., Competitive sustained exercise in humans, lymphokine activated killer cell activity, and glutamine — an intervention study, *Eur. J. Appl. Physiol.*, 78, 448, 1998.
41. Rowbottom, D.G., Keast, D., Garcia-Webb, P., and Morton, A.R., Training adaptation and biological changes among well-trained male triathletes, *Med. Sci. Sports Exerc.*, 29, 1233, 1997.
42. Nehlsen-Canarella, S.L., Fagoaga, O.R., Nieman, D.C., Henson, D.A., Butterworth, D.E., Bailey, E., Warren, B.J., and Davis, J.M., Carbohydrate and the cytokine response to 2.5 hours of running, *J. Appl. Physiol.*, 82, 1662, 1997.
43. Nieman, D.C., Henson, D.A., Garner, E.B., Butterworth, D.E., Warren, B.J., Utter, A., Davis, J.M., Fagoaga, O.R., and Nehlsen-Cannarella, S.L., Carbohydrate affects natural killer cell redistribution but not activity after running, *Med. Sci. Sports Exerc.*, 29, 1318, 1997.
44. Nieman, D.C., Fagoaga, O.R., Butterworth, D.E., Warren, B.J., Utter, A., Davis, J.M., Henson, D.A., and Nehlsen-Canarella, S.L., Carbohydrate supplementation affects blood granulocyte and monocyte trafficking but not function after 2.5 hours of running, *J. Appl. Physiol.*, 82, 1385, 1997.
45. Henson, D.A., Nieman, D.C., Parker, J.C., Rainwater, M.K., Butterworth, D.E., Warren, B.J., Utter, A., Davis, J.M., Fagoaga, O.R., and Nehlsen-Canarella, S.L., Carbohydrate supplementation and the lymphocyte proliferative response to long endurance running, *Int. J. Sports Med.*, 19, 574, 1998.
46. Nieman, D.C., Nehlsen-Canarella, S.L., Fagoaga, O.R., Henson, D.A., Utter, A., Davis, J.M., Williams, F., and Butterworth, D.E., Influence of mode and carbohydrate on the cytokine response to heavy exertion, *Med. Sci. Sports Exerc.*, 30, 671, 1998.
47. Nieman, D.C., Nehlsen-Canarella, S.L., Fagoaga, O.R., Henson, D.A., Utter, A., Davis, J.M., Williams, F., and Butterworth, D.E., Effects of mode and carbohydrate on the granulocyte and monocyte response to intensive prolonged exercise, *J. Appl. Physiol.*, 84, 1252, 1998.
48. Mitchell, J.B., Pizza, F.X., Paquet, B.J., Davis, B.J., Forrest, M.B., and Braun, W.A., Influence of carbohydrate status on immune responses before and after endurance exercise, *J. Appl. Physiol.*, 84, 1917, 1998.
49. Calder, P.C., Fat chance of immunomodulation, *Immunol. Today*, 19, 244, 1998.
50. Tvede, N., Heilmann, C., Halkjaer Kristensen, J., and Pedersen, B.K., Mechanisms of B-lymphocyte suppression induced by acute physical exercise, *J. Clin. Lab. Immunol.*, 30, 169, 1989.
51. Pedersen, B.K., Tvede, N., Klarlund, K., Christensen, L.D., Hansen, F.R., Galbo, H., Kharazmi, A., and Halkjaer Kristensen, J., Indomethacin *in vitro* and *in vivo* abolishes post-exercise suppression of natural killer cell activity in peripheral blood. *Int. J. Sports Med.*, 11, 127, 1990.
52. Benquet, C., Krzystyniak, K., Savard, R., and Guertin, F., Modulation of exercise-induced immunosuppression by dietary polyunsaturated fatty acids in mice, *J. Tox. Environ. Health*, 43, 225, 1994.

53. Cannon, J.G., Fiatarone, M.A., Meydani, M., Gong, J., Scott, L., Blumberg, J.B., and Evans, W.J., Aging and dietary modulation of elastase and interleukin-1 beta secretion. *Am. J. Physiol.*, 268, R208, 1995.

54. Johnson, J.A., Griswold, J.A., and Muakkassa, F.F., Essential fatty acids influence survival in sepsis, *J. Trauma.*, 35, 128, 1993.

55. Babior, B.M., Oxidants from phagocytes: agents of defense and destruction, *Blood*, 64, 959, 1984.

56. Hemila, H., Vitamin C and the common cold, *Br. J. Nutr.*, 67, 3, 1992.

57. Peters, E.M., Goetzsche, J.M., Grobbelaar, B., and Noakes, T.D., Vitamin C supplementation reduces the incidence of post-race symptoms of upper-respiratory-tract infection in ultramarathon runners, *Am. J. Clin. Nutr.*, 57, 170, 1993.

58. Peters, E.M., Campbell, A., and Pawley, L., Vitamin A fails to increase resistance to upper respiratory infection in distance runners, *S. Afr. J. Sports. Med.*, 7, 3, 1992.

59. Nieman, D.C., Henson, D.A., Butterworth, D.E., Warren, B.J., Davis, J.M., Fagoaga, O.R., and Nehlsen-Canarella, S.L., Vitamin C supplementation does not alter the immune response to 2.5 hours of running, *Int. J. Sports Nutr.*, 7, 173, 1997.

60. Nielsen, H.B., Secher, N.H., Kappel, M., and Pedersen, B.K., N-acetylcysteine does not affect the lymphocyte proliferation and natural killer cell activity response to exercise. *Am. J. Physiol*, 275, R1227, 1998.

61. Cannon, J.G., Meydani, S.N., Fielding, R.A., Fiatarone, M.A., Meydani, M., Farhangmehr, M., Orencole, S.F., Blumberg, J.B., and Evans, W.J., Acute phase response in exercise. II. Associations between vitamin E, cytokines, and muscle proteolysis, *Am. J. Physiol.*, 260, R1235, 1991.

62. Kasama, T.K., Kobayashi, T., Fukushima, M., Tabata, M., Ohno, I., Negishi, M., Ide, H., Takahashi, T., and Niwa, Y., Production of interleukin 1-like factor from human peripheral blood monocytes and polymorphonuclear leukocytes by superoxide anion: the role of interleukin–1 and reactive oxygen species in inflamed sites, *Immunol. Immunopathol.*, 53, 439, 1989.

63. Davies, K.J.A., Packer, I.., and Brooks, G.A., Free radicals and tissue produced by exercise, *Biochem. Biophys. Res. Commun.*, 107, 1198, 1982.

64. Meydani, S.N., Meydani, M., Blumberg, J.B., Leka, L.S., Siber, G., Loszewski, R., Thompson, C., Pedrosa, M.C., Diamond, R.D., and Stollar, B.D., Vitamin E supplementation and *in vivo* immune response in healthy elderly subjects, *JAMA*, 277, 1380, 1997.

Index